Psychology for Midwives

Psychology for Midwives

Ruth Paradice

Quay
Books

Mark Allen
Publishing Ltd

Quay Books Division, Mark Allen Publishing Limited, Jesses Farm,
Snow Hill, Dinton, Wiltshire, SP3 5HN

British Library Cataloguing-in-Publication Data
A catalogue record is available for this book

© Mark Allen Publishing Ltd 2002
ISBN 1 85642 040 X

Printed in the UK by Cromwell Press, Trowbridge, Wiltshire

Contents

Acknowledgements

I want to thank my husband Richard Clements who encouraged me to write the book and then provided me with practical support that gave me the time to write. I also want to thank my parents Charles and Val Paradice who have always encouraged me to achieve my full potential and have been so proud of everything I have accomplished. Mary Stewart gave me a great deal of help with the first drafts of the chapters on birth and loss. This came at a crucial time, when my life was so busy that I would have given up on the book without her input. I must also thank Tamzin Ewers and Binkie Mais at Quay Books, Mark Allen Publishing Limited for being prepared to wait so long before getting the book into print. They have been very patient. Most importantly, I want to acknowledge the midwifery students who attended the University of the West of England while I was lecturing there. Without their positive response to my teaching, their willingness to engage in discussion and their passion for their profession this book would never have come into existence.

Ruth Paradice
March 2002

Introduction

This book is the culmination of many years spent teaching psychology courses to health professionals. During this time my involvement with students studying a variety of courses related to health such as physiotherapy, radiography, health visiting, nursing, district nursing and, of course, midwifery has convinced me of the usefulness of psychology in helping students to develop their professional practice and gain a fuller understanding both of themselves and of the people they interact with in their day-to-day work. However, there are few textbooks available that bring together those aspects of psychological theory that are particularly useful for individual professional groups. At the beginning of her book the *Psychology of Pregnancy and Childbirth*, Lorraine Sherr makes this point when she argues that the academic discipline of psychology is not always made available to those health professionals who would find it useful:

> *... much of the (psychological) knowledge is locked up within the body of psychology and rarely emerges from ivory towers into the labour wards.*

> (Sherr, 1995, p. 4)

I hope to make psychology accessible to midwives by bringing together in one volume aspects of psychological theory that I believe are relevant and useful for midwifery practice.

The first chapter provides the reader with a very brief introduction to psychology. The various 'schools of thought' are described and the way psychologists obtain information about human behaviour is also discussed. I appreciate that this has the effect of throwing you in at the deep end, particularly if you have not done any psychology before, but I feel that it is important to give the reader a general overview of the subject as many people have misconceptions about what psychology is and what psychologists do. This misunderstanding is reflected in people's reactions when you tell them that you are a psychologist. The conversation (condensed for the purposes of this introduction) usually goes something like this:

Them:	*Hello, my name's John. Pleased to meet you.*
Me:	*Hi, I'm Ruth.*
Them:	*What do you do for a living, Ruth?*
Me:	*Well, I'm a psychologist.*
Them:	(Taking two steps away from me) *Oh.*

Sometimes that is the end of the conversation, and John goes off to find someone less threatening to talk to, but occasionally it continues:

Them:	*So,* (nervous laugh) *are you going to psycho-analyse me then? I'd better be careful what I say!*
Me:	*Well, actually I'm not qualified to psychoanalyse you, I teach developmental and social psychology at a university.*
Them:	(disappointed now) *Oh!*

I cannot tell you how many times I have had this conversation with people and nearly all of my colleagues have had similar experiences. So, after reading the first chapter of this book, you should be in no doubt about what psychologists are trying to do (mostly not psychoanalyse people). It will also help to set the rest of the book into the context of psychology as a whole. You will find that I rely far more heavily on social psychology than developmental psychology and hardly touch on cognitive psychology at all. Reading this chapter should enable you to understand why some aspects of psychology are more relevant to midwives and midwifery practice than others.

Of course, it is quite possible to omit this chapter altogether if you already have some knowledge of psychology.

How this book is organised

The book is divided into two sections. The first part discusses topics which are particularly relevant to the practice of the midwife. The focus is on the midwife gaining a fuller understanding of the psychology of the environment in which she works and of her own psychological responses to this; although mothers and babies are brought into the picture they are not the main focus. *Chapter 1* provides a brief introduction to psychology for those who know little about the different subject areas that make up the discipline. This chapter aims to help the reader to locate the content of the rest of the book within psychology as a whole. The next four chapters focus specifically on the midwifery context. *Chapter 2* considers how wider social forces, such as social influence can affect the work of the midwife and *Chapter 3* discusses the ways in which prejudice can influence relationships. *Chapter 4* looks at social attribution and discusses how this can influence the midwife. The final chapter in the first section looks at the importance of communication and communication skills in midwifery practice. In the second part of the book the focus shifts to the mother/baby dyad and they now become the main subject. We can see it almost as a figure-ground illusion. The midwife, mother and baby are in the frame throughout the book, but in the earlier chapters the midwife is fully in focus while the mother and baby reside in the background. This reverses in the second half of the book, where the mother and baby take centre stage. The chapters in this section follow a logical sequence beginning with pregnancy and following through to the period after childbirth. *Chapter 6* looks at pregnancy, *Chapter 7* considers labour, *Chapter 8* discusses early infancy, *Chapter 9* the postnatal period and *Chapter 10* loss and bereavement.

I have included topics which I believe are particularly relevant to midwifery practice and have tried to make the book accessible by using as little jargon as possible and by illustrating each chapter with examples taken from either midwifery practice or other healthcare settings. I hope you find it interesting, useful and enjoyable.

Ruth Paradice
December, 2001

Section 1:
Theoretical perspectives

1

What is psychology about?

Psychology is a relatively new science that began to be accepted as a separate discipline at the end of the nineteenth century. It developed out of philosophy and was also influenced by the biological sciences, particularly physiology. A good, simple working definition of psychology is, 'the scientific study of behaviour' (Glassman, 2000).

The two key words in this definition are scientific and behaviour and a closer examination of what psychologists understand these words to mean will help clarify what psychology is.

Most psychologists would agree that the subject matter of psychology is the study of behaviour, although they do not always agree about which aspects of behaviour are regarded as being appropriate for analysis. For example, the group of psychologists known as behaviourists believes that only behaviour that can be observed should be studied; they make no inferences about what their subjects are thinking or feeling. This contrasts with cognitive psychologists who devote their work entirely to the study of mental processes. For these psychologists the word behaviour would include thinking, perception, memory and emotion. They use observable behaviour such as problem-solving and memory tests to test hypotheses about the way the brain carries out these activities. Other psychologists would extend the use of the word behaviour to include the study of the behaviour of animals. Although not all psychologists agree, taken as a whole, the word behaviour in psychology must encompass actions (observable behaviour), mental processes (unobservable behaviour) and the behaviour of animals.

While there are differences among psychologists about the definition of the word behaviour, almost all psychologists would agree that as a discipline psychology attempts to be scientific. This means that systematic methods of observation and analysis are used to carry out psychological studies and draw conclusions about the underlying **causes** of behaviour. Psychologists do not make statements about behaviour simply because it is something that they believe or because it seems like common sense, they design experiments using precise scientific methods in order to discover whether the ideas they have about human behaviour are accurate. Sometimes these experiments are carried out in the laboratory and sometimes they are done outside in more natural settings, but they are always set up carefully so that the results that are obtained can be regarded as reliable and accurate. Statistical methods are then used to analyse the results to show whether they could have been obtained by chance or are genuinely due to the changes made during the experiment.

Of course, the use of this scientific method is not without its drawbacks, particularly when you are trying to study people. Many experiments that psychologists might like to do are impossible because they are unethical and experiments that are done in the laboratory are frequently criticised because they are not representative of a 'normal' situation. On the other hand, experiments that are carried out in the field sometimes yield such complex data that it is difficult to make sense of the results. Other problems arise because of the nature of the subject matter: people who participate in psychology experiments are not passive, they are interested in what is happening and they may try to change their behaviour in order to do what they think the experimenter wants, or they may try to do the opposite in order to spoil the experiment, or they may simply not behave normally because they are conscious of being observed. The complexity of the nature of human behaviour is such that it is often difficult to make general statements about what people will do in particular situations. Although this can make psychology experiments frustrating, at the same time it makes the subject fascinating and exciting. A fuller explanation of what is meant by 'the scientific method' is given in the second half of this chapter.

Despite these difficulties psychologists have accumulated quite a large body of knowledge about human behaviour. We do not yet have the complete picture, and perhaps we never will, but there are still many things that psychologists do know and this knowledge can be usefully applied for the health professional.

The main approaches in psychology

As we have already seen, within the discipline of psychology there are several branches that take different views of how behaviour is best explained. What follows is a brief description of each of these approaches (see Glassman, 2000 for a fuller account).

The biological approach

Two assumptions underpin this approach, firstly, that all behaviour has a physiological base and secondly, that behaviour can be genetically inherited. We can trace the roots of the first assumption back to the philosophical ideas of materialism (for an interesting account of materialism and other aspects of Western philosophy see Gaarder, 1995) and the second to the theories of Charles Darwin. Scientists working within this paradigm explore cause and effect relationships between behaviour and physiology. For example, pain felt by a woman in labour would be explained in terms of the physiological mechanisms that influence the pain response. The role of other, non-biological factors, such as the strangeness of the environment, the woman's level of anxiety or her past experiences would be acknowledged, but probably not emphasised.

In the minds of people in contemporary society there would be no doubt that the brain controls our behaviour or that it is the seat of our personality. We know that we would not be fundamentally different if we had to have a heart or a liver transplant, but a brain transplant would be impossible. The self, as we experience it, would disappear and cease to exist, along with our brain. It was not always so. In the ancient world there was heated debate about the location of the soul within the body and it was not until the middle of the eighteenth century that scientists began to argue that the mind and the soul were one and the same thing and were both located in the brain. This new concept, which went against the teaching of the church, was not finally accepted as a fact until the middle of the nineteenth century when more and more evidence made it impossible to think otherwise.

Just as we now acknowledge that the brain has a major influence on our behaviour, we also accept that many characteristics are controlled by the genes that we inherit from our parents and we understand the mechanisms by which simple characteristics, such as eye colour and height are passed on from one generation to the next. Within the biological approach, the debate about heritability has become more complex and now centres around how much of our behaviour is controlled genetically and how much is due to the environment. This has become known as the nature/nurture debate and is well illustrated by the arguments concerning the heritability of intelligence.

Francis Galton (1822–1911), a cousin of Charles Darwin, was one of the first people to suggest that we inherit our intelligence from our parents. Galton noted that intelligent people frequently produced intelligent children but he failed to take the environment into the equation at all. He did not consider that clever parents might well provide a rich and stimulating environment that would enhance the intellectual capacities of their offspring. Since Galton's time there has been an ongoing debate about this issue with varying results but, with extensive research on identical twins (who share exactly the same genetic constitution), there is a gradually emerging consensus about the relative contributions of inheritance and environment on intelligence. The nature of the interaction between genetic inheritance and the environment is still a topic of heated debate (Plomin, 2001; Rose, 2001).

Plomin (1995) is critical of those who seek to advance simple theories of genetic determinism. The idea that one gene is responsible for complex behaviour such as intelligence or even homosexuality is just not tenable. Such simplistic theorising is dangerous and inaccurate because genetic influence rarely accounts for more than half the variance in any population. The evidence is strongly suggestive that while heredity is of crucial importance the environment 'modifies' the influence of our genetic inheritance in complex and subtle ways. The challenge for psychologists is to untangle the interactions between nature and nurture so that those significant features of the environment that influence human behaviour can be better understood.

Some critics have argued that the biological approach is reductionist, that it reduces behaviour down to its basic components and that this simplifies things too much. In general, the biological approach does tend to take a somewhat mechanistic view of behaviour and because it focuses on the internal workings of the brain and nervous system, fails to consider the complex factors outside the individual that could be influential. This book only refers to the biological approach in the chapter on birth (*Chapter 7*), where we find that even in an area that would appear to be explicable at the physical level, environmental factors cannot be ignored.

Psychoanalytic psychology

Sigmund Freud (1856–1939) is the undisputed founding father of psychoanalytic psychology. His theories about the workings of the mind were revolutionary when they were first published and they began a completely new school of thought within the discipline of psychology. Although Freud's ideas are complex, it is possible to distil them down into those components that have been most influential in changing how we think about the human mind and behaviour. There are three aspects of Freudian theory that have had a major impact on contemporary thinking.

Firstly, Freud believed that a large part of the mind is inaccessible to us and he called this the **unconscious**. Under normal circumstances we have no way of knowing what the unconscious part of our mind contains but occasionally **dreams**, errors and **slips of the tongue** give us clues about its contents. Even then we need a skilled interpreter (a psychoanalyst) to help us make sense of them. Freud believed that we use what he called **defence mechanisms** to bury thoughts and feelings that are threatening or unacceptable to us in the unconscious. Unfortunately, we are rarely able to bury things completely and they have a nasty habit of influencing our behaviour in subtle and often unhelpful ways, expressing themselves as **neuroses** and other **maladaptive behaviours**. The purpose of **psychoanalysis** is to help the client to understand the elements of the unconscious that are affecting behaviour and this insight is believed to be enough to reduce or even eradicate the problem.

Secondly, Freud argued that what happens to us as children influences our adult behaviour. Our relationships with others, particularly our parents, continues to have an impact on us throughout life and traumatic childhood experiences can have damaging effects that extend into adulthood. Although there were other writers before Freud who highlighted childhood as an important and informative period of life, it was Freud who established the idea that childhood experiences link directly with adult behaviour. This concept has now become so entrenched in everyday thinking that it is hard to imagine that childhood experiences do not influence adult behaviours; although some theorists have argued that the relationship is not a simple one of cause and effect (Sameroff, 1989; Emde and Spicer, 2000) and is better seen as a series of transactions between the individual and the social environment in which they are growing up.

Thirdly, Freud shocked Victorian society by claiming that the main drive in life is a sexual one and he argued that children are sexual too. Freud also believed that sexual frustrations lead to neurotic and abnormal patterns of behaviour. This emphasis on sexuality was a complete departure from any other ideas that had gone before and although psychoanalytic writers who followed Freud argued that he attached too much importance to sexual behaviour, Freud's theory fundamentally changed our ideas about the significance of human sexuality.

Many other theorists have since followed in the psychoanalytic tradition, adapting Freud's theories to fit in with their own ideas about the human condition. Two of the most well known of these are Jung and Adler but others include Erikson, Fromm, Jones, Horney, Klein, Anna Freud, Bowlby and Winnicott. This book does not draw heavily on the ideas of psychoanalysis although, as indicated, many of the major concepts are now endemic in our thinking and are difficult to avoid. For the interested reader a fuller account of Freud's theory and many of the others mentioned can be found in Sayers (1991).

Behaviourism

This branch of psychology was being developed at about the same time as psychoanalytic psychology but it takes a radically different approach to the understanding of human behaviour. Whereas psychoanalysis looks within the mind to gain insight, behaviourism relies totally on observable behaviour and makes no attempt to analyse the contents of the 'black box', that is, what is going on inside the head. Behavioural psychologists argue that as behaviour is the only aspect of human activity that can be observed and described, it alone is open to scientific study. Anything that goes on within the mind can only be inferred from behaviour and is therefore not accessible to analysis.

The first psychologist who could be called a behaviourist was Edward L Thorndike (1874–1949). He noted that animals tend to learn by forming an association between a response and what happens immediately afterwards. Positive consequences tend to increase behaviour while negative consequences have the effect of reducing behaviour. For example, if an animal eats food and then vomits, the animal will learn to avoid that food by associating the food with an unpleasant experience. This relationship between behaviour and what follows came to be known as *The Law of Effect*.

Thorndike's ideas, although simple, were not without their problems, one of which was that he did not make it clear what constituted a positive or negative consequence. Another behaviourist, John B Watson (1878–1958) tried to address this by suggesting that behaviour is motivated by biological drives such as hunger and thirst. Anything which reduces these drives may be regarded as a positive consequence and will tend to increase the behaviour; events which do not reduce the drive or produce unpleasant consequences are negative. Consequences, which reduce a drive immediately, are **primary reinforcers**, so food for a hungry animal would fall into this category. Watson also believed that certain events could become **secondary reinforcers** by association with primary reinforcers. An example might be helpful here. Your pet cat learns through association that food reduces the unpleasant **primary drive** of hunger. The food is the primary reinforcer but as the person who always supplies the food you become associated with the reduction of hunger and thus become a secondary reinforcer, reinforcing in your own right. This explains (I think) why my cat wants to sit on my lap all the time, even when it is not at all convenient!

Perhaps the most famous behaviourist, Burrhus F Skinner (1904–1990) argued we do not really need the concept of drive to explain behaviour. Skinner claimed that if any behaviour that is in an animal's repertoire (he called these operants) is followed by an event that is rewarding then that behaviour will be repeated. So, if a hungry animal bites someone and is then given food, this will increase the biting behaviour. It follows that if you reward your dog (or your child) after they have behaved in a way that pleases you this will have the effect of increasing that behaviour, however, it is important that the reward follows immediately after the behaviour that you wish to increase. Any delay will reduce the effectiveness of the reinforcement. This basic principle underpins all animal training techniques and many behaviour modification programmes aimed at people.

Skinner's theory is known as **operant conditioning**. A Russian physiologist called Ivan Pavlov (1849–1936) developed the theory of **classical conditioning**. Again this is related to the idea of forming associations between two events but this time the associations are formed between naturally occurring biological reflexes and external events. Working with salivation in dogs, Pavlov noticed that the animals would salivate not only when they were eating food but also beforehand when they saw the experimenter bringing the bowl to them. Pavlov wondered whether dogs would learn to associate other unrelated stimuli to food and therefore salivate, so every time he gave the dogs food he also rang a bell. After many pairings of food and bell, Pavlov found that dogs would salivate when they heard the bell alone even when food was not given. We can observe this response in ourselves; just think for a moment about eating some kind of food that you enjoy, now think about your mouth. Are you salivating?

Pavlov called the naturally occurring reflex the **unconditioned response** (or UCR). In this example, the UCR is salivation. The food is the **unconditioned stimulus** (or UCS). The bell is the **conditioned stimulus** (CS) and salivation to the bell is the **conditioned response** (CR). **Classical conditioning** has been used to explain how people develop **phobias**. In this case we have associated the natural response of fear with a stimulus which is not intrinsically fearful. Various therapies are based on the idea of trying to break this association.

The major criticism of **behaviourism** is that, while it may be adequate for explaining animal behaviour, it does not take into account the complexity and unpredictability of human behaviour. A large part of human experience is tied up with experiences that are 'in the head'. **Emotions**, **feelings** and thoughts all influence our behaviour, so surely it is too simplistic to claim that we are controlled purely by environmental stimuli? Skinner would argue that internal states are:

> *... scientifically unknowable, and in any case do not **cause** behaviour: Thinking about something before doing it is simply **correlated** with the observable behaviour.*

> (Glassman, 2000, p. 145, author's emphasis)

Despite this criticism, behaviourism has influenced our thinking about human behaviour considerably. Behaviourist principles affect us all in our everyday life, even if it is only in terms of giving the dog a biscuit when he does something 'good'. Although there is no chapter in this book that takes a primarily behaviourist approach, we can hardly deny its existence and we will find that it often creeps in when we are least expecting it.

Humanistic psychology

While psychoanalytic psychology takes a rather pessimistic view of humanity, the humanistic approach regards people in a very positive light. Human nature is seen as being essentially good and motivated to develop in the direction of self-growth. Humanists argue that we are often prevented from achieving this positive self-development or self-actualisation (becoming everything one is capable of becoming) by life circumstances and by our upbringing.

The two most well known humanistic psychologists were Abraham Maslow (1908–1970) and Carl Rogers (1902–1987). Maslow suggested that there is a **hierarchy of needs** (*Figure 1.1*). Every individual seeks to fulfil these needs but more basic needs must be fulfilled first. Needs at the lower levels of the hierarchy have to be met before a person can move on to higher order needs. The hierarchical nature of needs means that we are often held back from developing our full potential, for example, we cannot consider meeting our needs for love and belongingness if safety and physiological needs remain unsatisfied.

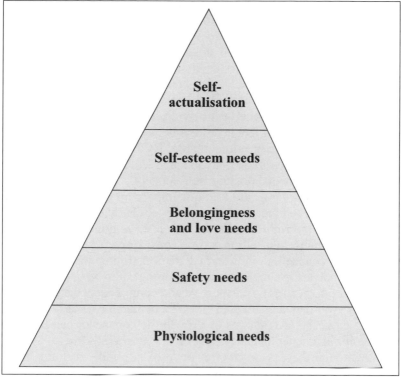

Figure 1.1: Maslow's Hierarchy of Needs (Maslow, 1971)

The four needs at the lower end of the hierarchy are regarded by Maslow as deficiency needs, that is, in each case something is missing which has to be supplied before we can move on. If we were cold and hungry we would have to find shelter and warmth before moving to the next stage in the hierarchy. Self-actualisation is the only need that is described as a growth need. Maslow believed that although everyone is capable of **self-actualisation**, very few people achieve this level of personal development, most of us are held back by our other needs.

Carl Rogers also took the view that everyone has the potential for positive self-growth and he called this the **actualising tendency**. He argued that this was a basic human motivation that influenced every human being, however, many of us are prevented from achieving our full potential because of the way that we are brought up. Rogers believed that everyone wants to feel that they are loved; we enjoy and seek attention and praise from others, particularly our parents. He described this as a need for **positive regard**. Unfortunately, when we are growing up most of us only receive positive regard when we behave in ways that are acceptable to our parents. In other words, we receive **conditional positive regard**; that is, praise and rewards are conditional upon us doing what our parents consider 'right'. We quickly learn that we do not receive positive regard for just being ourselves. Rogers argued that in order to reach one's full potential you have to receive unconditional positive regard from significant others and to feel loved by them even if your behaviour is considered to be socially unacceptable. By receiving unconditional positive regard it is possible to stay in touch with one's true feeling and maintain an accurate and positive self-concept.

Rogers' theory has had a major impact on counselling theory because he believed that the actualising tendency exists throughout life and under the right conditions it is always possible to achieve self-growth. In the counselling setting **conditions for growth** can be met by the counsellor or therapist demonstrating three qualities. Unconditional positive regard, **empathy** or the ability to understand the problems from the client's perspective and **congruence**; the counsellor is exactly who they are and does not hide behind a role or facade. By meeting these three conditions of growth the counsellor can help the client achieve a better understanding of who they really are.

Although there is no chapter devoted explicitly to humanistic psychology, the approach is implicit throughout much of this book as the conditions for growth can be applied beneficially in midwifery practice. If you are able to give your client unconditional positive regard, show empathy and be yourself then this will aid the establishment of a good relationship which can have further benefits for mother, baby and midwife. The humanistic approach is touched upon in the chapter on communication (*Chapter 5*).

Cognitive psychology

This approach is the opposite of behaviourism in that its subject matter deals almost exclusively with what goes on inside the 'black box'. While cognitive psychologists do not deny that stimuli produce responses they argue that **mental processes** come in-between the stimuli and the response. In other words, we think about a stimulus before we act. Because these mental processes come between stimuli and response they are called **mediators** and include problem solving, memory, forgetting, perception, learning and language.

Cognitive psychologists adhere strictly to the scientific method and most of the research in this area has been laboratory based. Of course, it is impossible for us physically to get inside the mind so it is assumed that behaviour provides the observer with clues about how the mind processes information. For example, we can develop an understanding of how memory works by giving people memory tasks and drawing conclusions based on their performance. From this information models of memory have been developed. These models do not necessarily map onto actual structures within the brain, but simply provide us with a means of understanding, describing and making sense of memory processes.

Social psychology

This branch of psychology focuses on behaviour in social situations and examines how people interact with each other and how they are influenced by groups. Social psychology tends to be generic in its approach in that it uses ideas from other areas of psychology (such as behaviourism and cognitive psychology) and a variety of methods have been used from observation to laboratory-based experiments.

The underlying philosophy of this approach is that not only are people social by nature but that their behaviour is affected by others in complex, but predictable ways. Social psychologists believe that although we like to think of ourselves as individuals, we make sense of our behaviour by comparing ourselves with others. Many social situations that we find ourselves in are ambiguous and we look to others for guidance on how we should behave. If we find that other people are doing the same as us, then we feel more comfortable about our own behaviour. An experiment by Schacter and Singer (1962) illustrates how we may even interpret our emotions by using others as social referents. Three groups of subjects were given an injection of adrenaline, which increases the heart rate and produces a state of arousal. One group was told what physical symptoms the drug would produce, a second group was told that the drug would produce numbness, itching and headaches and the third group was given no information at all. All the participants were then asked to wait in a room with one other person who was, in fact, a confederate of the experimenter. The confederate had been instructed to behave either in an angry or a happy way.

People in all the groups experienced arousal but only those in the first group correctly attributed it to the drug. Those in the other groups reported feeling angry or happy depending on the behaviour of the confederate. Here is an example where an ambiguous situation (subjects do not know why they feel aroused) is interpreted using the behaviour of another as a guide. Some level of arousal was necessary (a control group who had been injected with saline reported no emotion), but the *interpretation* of the internal state depended on the subject using the behaviour of a third party as a social referent.

In more recent years social psychologists have turned their attention to **social cognition** (see *Chapter 4*). Briefly, social cognition studies the perceptual processes that influence how we observe and make sense of the behaviour of others. It regards people as naive scientists who build **schemas** (or theories) to explain the social situations in which they find themselves. It is assumed that people are rarely passive but are actively trying to understand and interpret what they see. This branch of social psychology draws upon some of the insights made by cognitive psychology to enhance the understanding of social behaviour.

A large part of this book is devoted to social psychology, *Chapters 2, 3* and *4* deal with social influence, prejudice and stereotyping, attribution theory and attitudes. Throughout these chapters the theory is illustrated with examples that are relevant to health professionals in general and midwifery practice in particular.

Developmental psychology

Like social psychology, this approach uses a variety of methods to study development and draws on nearly all the other approaches in its efforts to explain how and why development occurs. Unlike social psychology, most of developmental psychology focuses on the individual and it is only in recent years that the influence of the social context on development has been recognised. Development may be defined as:

> *The process by which a child or foetus and more generally an organism (human or animal), grows and changes throughout its life-span.*

> (Smith *et al*, 1998, p. 7)

The aim of studying human developmental psychology is to describe the changes that occur, and explain how and why they are happening in the hope of discovering aspects of change that are universal in all humans.

During the life-span of any individual change is constantly taking place, we are never static, not only do we alter physically but our behaviour and thinking develop as we age. These changes do not progress at a uniform rate, there are times in life when change is very rapid and others when it is more gradual. Childhood and adolescence is the period of time when most rapid development is occurring and for this reason developmental psychologists have concentrated their investigations on the earlier years of the life-span.

The nature/nurture debate has always been influential in developmental psychology. Clearly, some aspects of development are due to maturation, the age at which a baby cuts its first tooth or a girl begins her periods are largely under biological control; while other aspects of development appear to be more influenced by the environment. One of the primary tasks of development psychologists has been to try to tease apart these two influences and calculate how much of any developmental change is due to biological mechanisms and how much is due to the environment. There has been a gradual shift in emphasis over the last few decades. Thirty years ago, the environment was felt to be the most important influence on development but more recently there has been a change in focus and biological factors are increasingly regarded as playing a major role. This sea of change can be seen in the research that has been done on the abilities of the new born (see *Chapter 8*). As methods of studying neonates become more sophisticated and more is learned about what newborns can actually do, it is coming to be accepted that many of their abilities must be biologically determined.

Psychology and the scientific method

From the very beginning, psychology has struggled to emulate the natural sciences in their use of the **scientific method**. I believe that there are two reasons for this: firstly, psychologists were anxious that psychology was accepted as a *bona fide* scientific discipline by other scientists and secondly, the complex nature of its subject matter meant that it was essential to use well established methodologies. Without these, experimental findings could not be regarded as either accurate or reliable.

Psychology has always aimed to discover and describe **universal** laws of behaviour that would be applicable to all people in all situations, and the emphasis has been on **empirical** (based on empiricism, ie. the philosophical notion that all behaviour is learned) **research**. This means that psychological research is based on making observations of behaviour. These observations cannot be made any-old-how; simply watching people at a party cannot be called empirical research, but must be made objectively and be related to a particular theoretical perspective.

Theories in psychology are derived using either **inductive** or **deductive reasoning**. In practice, these are two sides of the same coin and are often difficult to disentangle. Glassman (2000) explains the distinction succinctly:

> *Induction involves forming general principles from specific observations. The story of Isaac Newton discovering gravity by being hit by a falling apple is doubtless folklore. What is not folklore is that Newton saw a connection between falling apples and orbiting planets — that is, gravity was a general principle that could be used to link these observations. Deduction, by contrast, involves drawing specific conclusions from a set of general principles. For example, Freud believed that aggression is an innate drive that can be expressed in destructive behaviour. From this it follows that if someone commits murder, it is because of this innate drive.*

> (Glassman, 2000, p. 16)

Both types of reasoning can be used to generate theory, which is a set of general principles, and from theory one can use deductive reasoning to derive **hypotheses** that can be tested by making further observations. Scientific investigation is in a continuous state of flux and renewal; as hypotheses are tested, theories may be proved, disproved or modified to take into account the new information that becomes available. This is particularly true in psychological investigation where the complexity of the subject matter means that we rarely achieve a complete understanding of human behaviour.

Research methods

These can be broadly divided into experimental and non-experimental techniques. As the name implies, **experimental methods** often involve studies that are laboratory based but this is not always the case. By contrast, and just to confuse you, **non-experimental** techniques can be done in the laboratory. All of the methods that are discussed have both strengths and weaknesses. A good researcher attempts to choose a method that is appropriate for the question that is being asked and plan the research carefully so that any weaknesses inherent in the method are kept to a minimum.

Experimental methods

When we talk of methodologies that are experimental we are really talking about the way the study is done, rather than its location, although experiments often do take place in the laboratory. When a psychologist uses an experimental method she begins with a hypothesis, which is a prediction of what will happen in a given situation. As we have seen, the hypothesis is not something that is just plucked out of the air but is related to a particular theoretical approach. The researcher then attempts to control as much of the situation as possible. In this way she can be sure that the results obtained are due to the **variables** that have been manipulated in the experimental situation and not to other influences that have not been accounted for. An example is helpful in making sense of all of this. Let's imagine an hypothesis (derived from theory of course) that number of hours sleep is related to performance on a memory test. The more sleep you have the better your performance will be. To test this hypothesis a psychologist gathers together a number of subjects, and divides them into groups allowing different amounts of sleep to each group. The next day subjects are given a memory test and the results of the different groups are obtained, much to our psychologist's delight she finds that her hypothesis has been supported. The number of hours of sleep does appear to be related to performance on a memory test. In this experiment the variable that has been manipulated by the experimenter is the number of hours of sleep but can she exclude other explanations for her results?

The answer to the question is no because there are several flaws in this experiment which would indicate that the results cannot be relied upon. For example, how did the researcher measure hours of sleep? Some of the subjects might have fallen deeply asleep almost immediately, while others might have dozed for some time. Could these be equated? What about the subjects, were they representative of the population? Were all the subjects of a similar intelligence level? Were there differences in the amount of sleep needed by the subjects? In this fictional experiment, there were too many other variables apart from hours of sleep that the experimenter had not been able to regulate. In order to draw definite conclusions, it is crucial to design the experiment so that as many variables as possible are controlled and accounted for in the experimental design.

Hopefully, this example has demonstrated what psychologists mean by variables and how important it is that these are taken into consideration when designing an experiment. In reality, because psychologists are working with people it is impossible to control all variables. Conditions within a laboratory can be held constant, but other factors could always become **confounding variables**, that is variables that influence the results. To take a silly example, in the above experiment perhaps it was not hours of sleep that influenced the results but whether people ate Shredded Wheat or Sugar Puffs for their breakfast. Of course, this is highly unlikely to have an effect on the results, but there is always the possibility that a confounding variable influences the results in a way that could not have been predicted beforehand.

Non-experimental methods

A number of types of study fall into this category.

Observation

Using this method, the researcher does not attempt to influence the situation in any way but simply watches and notes behaviour. Sometimes there are particular behaviours that are being studied, but often the observation is carried out in an open way with the aim of 'finding out' what behaviours occur in which settings.

The disadvantage of observational methods is that the presence of the observer can influence what is observed. People's behaviour changes when they know that they are being watched. To avoid this problem, **participant observation** is sometimes used. This involves the researcher becoming a member of the group that is being studied and has the advantage that his or her presence becomes normal and is less likely to affect the outcome.

The strength of this method is that human behaviour is observed in natural environments and so it is more likely to be representative of what people really do. The drawback is that it is impossible for the researcher to describe every detail of complex human interactions and inevitably some of the richness is lost in the analysis.

Correlational studies

These involve finding out whether two pieces of information are related in either a positive or negative way. For example, a researcher might wish to test whether intelligence level is related to the number of GCSE passes gained by a student. If it was found that as intelligence increased then students gained more GCSE passes then this would indicate the existence of a **positive correlation**. If, however, GCSE passes fell as intelligence increased, then this would indicate a **negative correlation** between the two measures. There is a third possibility too, that there is no relationship at all between the measures.

The problem with correlational studies is that they only demonstrate that a relationship *exists* between two pieces of information. There is no way of indicating whether one variable *causes* the other. When it seems logical that two pieces of information should go together then there is a danger that we imply causality. In the above example it seems like common sense that intelligence would influence a student's success at exams, but with correlation we can only say that the two things are related.

Such correlational studies are often used in health settings and can prove misleading. Several years ago it was shown that there was a positive correlation between heart disease and levels of cholesterol in the blood. This led to health professionals suggesting that reducing the level of cholesterol would reduce the risk of heart disease. We now know that the picture is much more complicated and reducing levels of cholesterol does not necessarily reduce heart disease. It was wrongly assumed that the positive correlation between cholesterol levels and heart disease meant that high cholesterol levels caused heart disease. While we can say that cholesterol levels are implicated in heart disease, correlation does not allow us to go further than this.

Questionnaires

We are all familiar with questionnaires, they occur frequently in magazines and they are the stock in trade of the market researcher. For the psychologist or health professional they can provide a means of gaining a large quantity of data fairly quickly and easily. It is not difficult to send out hundreds (or thousands) of questionnaires and encompass a large cross-section of the population in one fell swoop. They are usually fairly easy to analyse because they either require simple 'yes', 'no' responses or involve scales where the respondent has to indicate the strength or weakness of their feelings about a particular question.

There are several disadvantages. Generally, responses to questionnaires lack depth. Because respondents are restricted to fairly simple answers, they are unable to give a full picture of their true feelings and often the response categories offered do not coincide with what the respondent would really like to say. Secondly, it is not uncommon for people to fall into response sets, that is, they continually choose the same answer for all the questions and do not reflect their true feelings. In the same vein, respondents sometimes attempt to work out what the researcher really wants to know and structure their answers accordingly and occasionally they answer in a way intended to deliberately mislead. All this adds up to the fact that one has to be cautious when drawing conclusions from questionnaires, and unless they are very carefully constructed they may not be the best way of finding out about people.

Interviewing

This has proved a popular method of obtaining data and is frequently used in healthcare settings. Broadly speaking, there are two types of interview technique. One involves using a structured interview in which questions are prescribed and there is little room for an individual to enlarge on his or her responses. The second involves a semi-structured method in which the researcher has a few key questions but the participant is encouraged to talk freely about their answers to these questions and develop their own line of thinking. This method provides a richer source of data but is more difficult to analyse because responses may not fall into fixed categories.

As with questionnaires, similar problems regarding the nature of responses arise. We assume that respondents are giving accounts that reflect their true feelings, opinions and attitudes but we cannot always be sure of this.

Analysis of structured interviews is reasonably straightforward and usually quantitative methods are used. Semi-structured interviews are generally analysed using qualitative methods.

A note about qualitative and quantitative methods of analysis

Raw, unanalysed data generally yields little useful information. Once you have carried out a study and have obtained your information, you have to do something with it. It is likely that as a health professional you are most familiar with quantitative methods of analysis, because these are the methods most favoured in medical research. Quantitative methods utilise statistics to simplify and make sense of data so that general conclusions can be drawn from them. More recently, some psychologists and researchers in the health field have been turning to qualitative methods because they believe that these allow us to understand human problems in greater depth. They argue that it is almost impossible to draw general conclusions about people based on relatively small samples which can never be representative of an entire population. Therefore, it is better to understand a small group well. It is impossible to give a full account of the pros and cons of qualitative methods of analysis here, but a good account can be found in Bannister *et al* (1994).

Conclusion

The Midwives Rules and Code of Practice (UKCC, 1998) describe the duties of the midwife. The emphasis in these documents is on the physical care of both mother and baby. As seen in *Changing Childbirth* (Department of Health [DoH], 1993) there is a growing recognition of the need for midwives to provide psychological care to women and their families as well. The aim of this book is to describe some of the complex issues that may affect women during pregnancy, labour and the early postpartum. It is hoped that a clearer understanding of the psychological component of these events in a woman's life will enable you to add to the skills that you already use to support women during a very significant period in their lives, empowering them to have the birth experience that they want.

Psychology has been characterised by some as an imprecise science. Indeed, health professionals who are used to the more definite answers provided by the 'harder' sciences sometimes find psychology difficult because it rarely seems to offer unilateral answers to problems, but rather provides several possible explanations for any given behaviour. While this can be frustrating, the truth is that situations involving human behaviour are extremely complex and there is hardly ever a simple answer but always a range of possible explanations.

While a knowledge of psychology does not always furnish us with definite, clear-cut answers to the human condition, it does enable the practitioner to have a fuller understanding of the complex forces that may be influential in any given situation. Such knowledge can help the health professional to work more empathetically with clients which should lead to a better outcome for both midwife and client.

Consider the situation of the midwife in the labour ward, helping a woman to give birth to her baby This is a situation that the midwife deals with every day of her working life and at first the circumstances may appear quite straightforward. Two individuals are engaged in the same task, both are hoping for the same outcome. If we look beneath the surface a little we find that the scenario is not as simple as may first appear. To begin with, both participants bring their own personal histories into the labour room and these histories may be related to the distant past or to a more recent past. For example, the mother may have a deep-seated fear of the pain of labour, which might make her frightened, tense and unable to relax; or she may have had a stillbirth that makes her very anxious about this labour. The midwife has perhaps had an argument with her partner before leaving for work that day and this could have left her feeling irritable or depressed, or she might be feeling anxious about her professional skills in dealing with this particular labour. Both past and recent histories will influence the way that the participants will respond.

Although both participants in this situation have common goals, mother and midwife have different concerns during labour. The mother may be anxious about coping with pain, she may have fears about her own health and the health of her baby, she may be worrying about other children left at home. In addition, she has to cope with being in a strange environment and may be feeling that she has little or no control over what happens to her. The midwife, on the other hand, has to balance her professional skills against her interpersonal skills which may sometimes be in conflict, particularly if the labour is complicated or the midwife finds it hard to feel sympathetic towards a certain woman.

As if this were not enough, the scenario is complicated further by the presence of other people. The midwife and mother are not alone, other people involved in the situation will have an effect on it. A woman's partner is likely to be present at the birth and he may be more or less supportive. Some women in labour feel as if they have to help their partner cope as well as give birth. Similarly, the midwife's actions and decisions may well be influenced by colleagues and this, in turn, will influence the way that she interacts with the mother.

In this superficially straightforward situation there are many layers that need to be understood at both an **interpersonal** and an **intrapersonal** level. Each individual who is involved will bring their own personal history into the situation and this will have an impact upon their expectations, behaviour and how they interact with others (intrapersonal). At the interpersonal level, the actors in our fictitious scenario will find that their behaviour is influenced by the other people involved and by the nature of the relationships they have with them. The final layer is the wider social context in which all of this is taking place; this will have an impact too. Hospital policy, the nature of the team and how they interact with each other, and the pregnant woman's own social background, will all contribute to the final outcome.

With so many factors involved in understanding the outcome it is hardly surprising that psychology cannot provide simple and straightforward answers to some of the problems that could arise in this setting. What psychology can do is to give the midwife insight to help her make sense of and understand the complex nature of the situation that she finds herself in. Ultimately this can help her deal with the situation in a way that will improve her professional practice and will have a beneficial outcome for herself and her client.

I believe that studying psychology should be of personal benefit to the health professional as well as benefiting the client. My years of contact with people involved in health has demonstrated vividly the stresses and strains that are inherent in this kind of work, and so this book is as much about gaining insight into one's own behaviour as it is about developing understanding of the client. Developing **reflective practice** is an important aspect of professional development and is a key feature of the chapters that follow, all of which look at psychological theory, both from the perspective of the client and the perspective of the midwife.

My work as a counsellor has also convinced me of the importance of seeing everyone as an individual, and considering how their own personal histories contribute to their behaviour in a particular situation. This is a view that is certainly endorsed by *Changing Childbirth* (DoH, 1993). Let me illustrate this with an example. In midwifery practice at the present time there is a general belief that male partners in the delivery room are a 'good thing'. While I have no doubt that the majority of women do find their partner supportive and are glad to have him present, this may not be true for everyone. A woman might have all kinds of reasons for not wanting her partner present but because of the prevailing norm that exists it may be difficult for her to voice her doubts. By the same token, many men may feel unable to refuse to be present at their wife's labour. There is certainly evidence to indicate that some men feel that they have been dragooned into the labour room and find the experience of seeing their partner in pain traumatic (Parke, 1996). It is my belief that clients need to be listened to so that their individual wishes can be understood. Pigeonholing should be avoided as much as possible.

What's in a name?

It is often difficult to know exactly what to call pregnant women. Patient seems wrong because women who are pregnant are not ill and do not wish to see themselves in this light. On the other hand, recent research has indicated that 'client' is not favoured by pregnant women themselves, who prefer to be referred to as either 'mother-to-be' or simply 'pregnant woman' (Batra and Lilford, 1996). It is hard to please everyone so in this book I tend to use a variety of terms including 'client' (sorry mums), 'pregnant women' and mothers. As much as possible I also try to avoid sexist terminology and refer as frequently to 'she' as 'he' wherever this is appropriate. I do refer to midwives as 'she' throughout the book because, although the number of male midwives is increasing, there are still relatively few in the profession, so I apologise in advance to any male midwives who may be reading this book and feel excluded.

References

Batra N, Lilford R (1996) Not clients, not consumers and definitely not maternants. *Eur J Obstet Gynaecol Reprod Biol* **64**: 197–9

Bannister P, Burman E, Parker I, Taylor M, Tindall C (1994) *Qualitative Methods in Psychology: A research guide*. Open University Press, Milton Keynes

Department of Health (1993) *Changing Childbirth: Report of the Expert Maternity Group*. HMSO, London

Emde R, Spicer P (2000) Experience in the midst of variation: New horizons for development and psychopathology. *Dev Psychopathol* **12**(3): 313–31

Gaarder J (1995) *Sophie's World*. Phoenix, London

Glassman WE (2000) *Approaches to Psychology*. 3rd edn. Open University Press, Milton Keynes

Maslow A (1971) *The Farther Reaches of Human Nature*. Penguin, Harmondsworth

Parke RD (1996) *Fatherhood*. Harvard University Press, Cambridge, Mass

Plomin R (1995) Genetics and children's experiences in the family. *J Child Psychol Psychiatry* **36**(1): 33–68

Plomin R (2001) Genetics and behaviour. *The Psychologist* **14**(3): 134–9

Rose S (2001) DNA is important — but only in its proper place. *The Psychologist* **14**(3): 144–5

Sameroff AJ (1989) Principles of development and psychopathology. In: Sameroff AJ, Emde RN, eds. *Relationship Disturbances in Early Childhood*. Basic Books, New York

Sayers J (1991) *Mothering Psychoanalysis*. Hamish Hamilton, London

Schacter S, Singer JE (1962) Cognitive, social and physiological determinants of emotional state. *Psychol Rev* **60**: 379–99

Sherr L (1995) *The Psychology of Pregnancy and Childbirth*. Blackwell, Oxford

Smith PK, Cowie H, Blades M (1998) *Understanding Children's Development*. 3rd edn. Blackwell, Oxford

United Kingdom Central Council for Nursing, Midwifery and Health Visiting (1998) *The Midwives Rules and Code of Practice*. UKCC, London

2

Social influence or — you do as you are told

Imagine that you are sitting in a meeting where a proposal is being discussed about a contentious issue with which you strongly disagree. It appears from the conversation that the other people in the group are in favour of the proposal. You feel that you must voice your concerns about the issue that is being discussed, but when you outline your objections there is silence from the others in the group. It seems that nobody else in the room agrees with your viewpoint and no one comes forward to support you. Later on a vote is taken on the issue; What do you do? Do you vote with your conscience, do you abstain, or do you go along with the feelings of the others in the group; after all, as no one agrees with your opinion perhaps you are wrong? Perhaps this is a familiar scenario and you have actually been confronted with this situation in the past and know how you behaved on that occasion. I suspect that whatever you do (or did) you will come out of the meeting feeling uncomfortable. For various reasons we find it difficult to express our own views when these appear to conflict with the opinions of everyone else. This chapter explores why this happens and considers the relevance of social influence to midwifery practice.

How do psychologists explain social influence?

Every day of our lives our behaviour is subtly influenced by the people who comprise the society in which we live. We all tend to wear similar clothes, we line up at the supermarket and wait to pay, we adhere to social rules of politeness often thanking people when they have hurt us (the dentist for example) or given us bad news and saying sorry when something is not our fault. Our lives are dominated by these social norms and in general we tend to go along with them and do what we believe that society expects of us. If you have ever been in a situation when you have flown in the face of social norms you will realise how difficult this is and how uncomfortable you feel.

Going along with what everyone expects is much easier than branching out and 'doing your own thing'. What is the explanation for this? In Western culture a high priority is placed on being your own person and making decisions that are right for you, and yet most of us find it extremely difficult to do this.

Human beings are social animals and generally prefer to live in groups. Very few people choose to live their lives isolated from the rest of society, most of us spend the greater part of our time involved in one group or another. As children we are part of the family group, later on we enter school and establish groups of friends and as adults we may join groups and societies and also become part of a group associated with the job that we do. Being a group member has many benefits for the individual. It provides us with companionship, fulfils our safety needs and helps us to feel that we 'belong'. It also validates our sense of self as we tend to seek out and associate with others who hold similar ideas and values and this helps to give us a sense of knowing who we are. The family group is particularly important for us when we are children as it provides nurturance and protection and basic training in the cultural norms of the society in which we live.

There is a price to pay for group membership. In order to function, all groups, however small, have to establish social norms. These are rules and regulations that group members need to follow if the group is to stay together as a unit. Social norms vary from group to group in both formality and flexibility. In some groups the norms are laid out as formal 'rules of membership'; in other groups, the norms are unwritten and are more adaptable to the needs of the group members. In either case, if a group member continually flies in the face of the group norms he or she will be 'encouraged' to adhere to the 'rules'. If the individual wishes to remain a member of that particular group then they will probably conform to the group pressure, however, if they continue to disregard the group norms they may eventually cease to be considered as members of that particular group and will be asked to leave. Alternatively, if an individual disagrees with group norms he or she may choose to leave the group and join another that fits better with their needs.

The pressure that we feel to 'fit-in' with others is called social influence and can been defined as (Van Avermaet, 1996, p. 488):

> *... a change in the judgements, opinions and attitudes of an individual as a result of being exposed to the judgements, opinions and attitudes of other individuals.*

Psychologists have questioned why we are so susceptible to this. One explanation is that we want to be liked and we fear that we will not be if we refuse to do what people ask of us. From childhood, we learn that being helpful and doing what others expect can cause them to like us (Baron and Byrne, 1996), and so we repeat this pattern into adulthood. This desire to be liked and fit in with other's expectations is known as **normative social influence** and often leads to **public compliance**; that is, the individual changes their behaviour to fit in with group norms, but doesn't really change their private opinions at all.

Another explanation is known as **informational social influence**. Most of us wish to behave in an appropriate manner and do things correctly, but social situations are often ambiguous and it is difficult to be sure that we are right. Under these circumstances we turn to others for information about the 'correct' thing to do. Imagine being at a very formal dinner where there are about five different sizes of knives and forks and several different wine glasses, you are not at all sure which of the pieces of cutlery should be used for the butter and you have no idea which of the glasses you should use for which wine. What do you do? My guess is that you surreptitiously look to the other guests and observe which cutlery and glasses they are using. Seeing that others are behaving in the same way reassures us that our own behaviour is acceptable. **Private acceptance** is said to have occurred if an individual changes their opinions and/or behaviour according to information obtained from others.

Monkey-see-monkey-do: conformity without pressure

So far we have considered social influence from the point of view of the individual who is subjected to it. But what about the other side of the coin — what of the situation where you might wish to encourage someone to conform? You may be horrified by this suggestion and you could be forgiven for regarding the use of techniques to induce conformity totally unethical. However, in the healthcare setting there are situations where conformity would be in the best interests of the client. For example, attendance at antenatal clinics is generally regarded as a helpful screening procedure, safeguarding the health of both mother and baby. Conformity to the 'norm' of attendance would be beneficial. Psychologists have studied the conditions under which people are more likely to conform and I think it is helpful to the midwife to have an understanding of them.

Conformity is far more likely when someone owes you a favour. There is a powerful social norm that obligates individuals to reciprocate behaviours that they have received from others, it follows that any individual will be more likely to comply with a request from you if you have done something helpful for them first (Cialdini, 1995). **Reciprocal concessions** occur when someone tones down an initially large request, this gives the impression that they have made compromises and it is more likely to produce compliance. This technique is frequently used by market stall hagglers when they ask way too much for an article and then climb down on the price. It gives the buyer the sense that the stall holder is really making a major concession. Some psychologists have described this method of inducing compliance as the **door-in-the-face technique**. Cialdini *et al* (1975) stopped students in the street and asked them if they would volunteer to counsel juvenile delinquents for two hours a week for two years. Not surprisingly, all of them refused. When the request was toned down and the students were asked to take juvenile delinquents on a two-hour visit to the zoo, 50% agreed. By contrast, only 17% of a control group who received no initial request but were only asked to take juvenile delinquents on a trip to the zoo, complied. In another experiment, Cialdini and Ascani (1976) asked people to participate in a long-term scheme for donating blood. Although most refused this request, 50% then agreed to donate blood on a one-off basis. Only 32% of those who had not been asked the larger request complied with the one-off donation of blood.

A similar method of inducing compliance is called the **foot-in-the-door technique**. This involves asking for a small favour, followed by a much larger request. Freedman and Fraser (1966) phoned homeowners and asked them to participate in a market research survey. Once people had agreed they were questioned about the brands of soap they used. Later the same homeowners were contacted again and asked to participate in a much bigger survey that involved teams of researchers making an inventory of all the cleaning products in their household. It was explained that the researchers would have to spend several hours in the home and would need permission to go into drawers and cupboards in order to carry out the inventory thoroughly. This is obviously a much larger request than the first, but 52.8% of people agreed. The compliance in a control group who received the large request without the initial smaller request was only 22.2% by comparison.

Compliance, conformity and obedience: three aspects of social influence

As well as attempting to understand what causes us to succumb to social influence, social psychologists have studied a number of situations in which social influence occurs. This has led to a description of three subtypes of social influence, namely: compliance, conformity and obedience.

Compliance

Compliance occurs when we behave in accordance with a request made by another person. Such requests can happen many times a day and more often than not we do what we have been asked. Only occasionally do we refuse. Sometimes compliance costs us very little and we get pleasure from doing something helpful for somebody else. Often we comply because we need to for our own purposes, refusing to sign a cheque for goods would mean that we would not receive the items that we wanted to buy. Every so often, we are asked to do something that we are not so happy with and saying no is often difficult unless we can think of a good excuse for refusing.

Our tendency to comply is often very strong. Milgram (1974) carried out a study in which confederates asked people on a busy commuter train if they would give up their seats. Confronted with a direct request it was surprising how many people agreed, even though the initial solicitation was quite unreasonable. People were prepared to give up their seats to an able-bodied man and stand in the aisle, just because they had been asked.

Conformity

A classic experiment by Asch (1956) illustrates the power of group pressure. Subjects were asked to take part in a visual discrimination task. The exercise was straightforward enough, they had to decide which of three comparison lines (labelled A, B and C) was equal in length to a target line. The judgement was not difficult to make, in all the trials it was fairly obvious which of the three comparison lines was the same as the target line (*Figure 2.1*). In the first experiment, Asch found that when subjects were tested alone they made very few errors. In fact, of the thirty-seven people tested in this condition, thirty-five made no errors at all and the remaining two subjects made three errors between them. This gives an error rate of 0.7% (Van Avermaet, 1996).

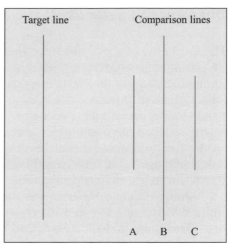

A very different picture emerged in a variation of the procedure. In this condition subjects were asked to do the same visual discrimination task with six other people who, unknown to the subject, were all confederates of the experimenter. The confederates and subject were seated in a semicircle and asked to make their judgements about line

Figure 2.1: Example of visual discrimination task shown to subjects in Asch's experiment

length, but the room was arranged so that the true subject gave his response after five of the confederates had given theirs. For the first few trials the confederates gave correct responses, but after a while began making predetermined errors. Asch was interested to know what people would do when subjected to this amount of social pressure. Would they deny the evidence of their own eyes? The results showed that although subjects did not conform on every occasion, they did on a significant number and the error rate rose to 37%. A huge leap from the 0.7% found in the control experiment.

Although in this example the confederates were not exerting social pressure in the sense of trying to persuade the one real subject to change his or her response, the effect was that the subject perceived social pressure and found it difficult to answer in a way that was contradictory to the responses being made by the other people in the group. The conclusion that we can draw from this experiment is that we are not comfortable when our opinion differs markedly from the opinions of others and under these circumstances we might either comply with the opinions being expressed by the group or seek out others whose opinions do agree with our own. This is an example of normative conformity where subjects change their response to fit in with the group, while knowing that the responses they give are, in fact, incorrect.

Obedience to authority

The third kind of social influence that has been described by social psychologists is obedience. Obedience occurs when we are told to do something by a person who is in a position of authority over us. This aspect of social influence has been studied in some detail by social psychologists because it has such potentially dangerous consequences when used by malign authority figures. In such regimes people have tortured or massacred others because they were carrying out the orders of those in authority over them, but obedience to authority can also occur in less dramatic situations.

Many years ago my sister was attending an antenatal clinic. The clinic was running late and many women were still waiting to be seen. The clinic midwife announced that if all the women took off their knickers while they were waiting it would help the doctor and speed things up. My sister (a psychology graduate) was the only one who refused to comply with the request. Shocking as it may seem now (I *think* antenatal clinics have changed) this vignette illustrates another aspect of conformity, that is, we are more likely to comply when we see other people doing the same. This is the principle behind much fund raising. If we see other people giving to charity then we are far more likely to follow suit; we are also more likely to comply with requests from people who we like or who we regard as friends. This brings us back to a point we began with, one of the reasons we conform is because we want people to like us and be seen to fit in.

The most well known study of obedience was done at Stanford University by a psychologist called Stanley Milgram (1963). Milgram had been influenced by Asch's experiments on conformity and believed that acts of atrocity such as those perpetrated against the Jews in World War II and in the My Lai massacre in Vietnam could be explained by social influence. He argued that the people who carried out such acts were not necessarily inhuman monsters, but were responding to the orders given to them by people in authority. He set up an experiment to test this idea.

Milgram put an advertisement in a local paper asking people to take part in an experiment on learning. On arrival at the laboratory subjects were introduced to another 'volunteer' who was in fact a confederate of the experimenter. They were told that they would play the part of either 'teacher' or 'learner' in the experiment and lots were drawn to see who would be the learner and who would be teacher. Although it seemed as if this was random it was in fact rigged so that the confederate of the experimenter was the learner and the true participant (the one who had responded to the newspaper advertisement) was the teacher.

The learning task was a lengthy list of word pairs such as nice-day, fat-neck; and this list of word pairs was read to the learner by the teacher, then both teacher and learner were taken into a small room where electrodes were attached to the arms of the learner. The experimenter explained that the learner would receive electric shocks for incorrect responses to the learning task. When asked if there were any questions the learner said that he had a heart condition and wanted to know whether the shocks would affect this. The experimenter explained that although the shocks would be painful they were harmless and both experimenter and subject left the room.

The teacher was then seated at a complicated switchboard that was described to him as an electric shock generator. Each switch was marked with the voltage it would deliver beginning at 15 volts and increasing by increments of 15 volts up to 450 volts. Labels on the switchboard gave an indication of the severity of the shock that would be delivered; 15–60 volts were described as slight shock, 75–120 volts as moderate shock; 135–180 volts as strong shock; 195–240 volts as very strong shock; 255–300 volts as intense shock; 315–360 volts as extremely intense shock; 375–420 volts as danger, severe shock and finally 425–450 volts simply as XXX. Teachers were told that they had to increase the shock administered to the learner by 15 volts for every incorrect answer given to the word pairs.

As the experiment progressed the learner began to complain about the pain of the shocks until eventually he was shouting to be let out of the room. The teacher was urged by the experimenter to continue the experiment, what Milgram wanted to know was how far people would go before they refused to continue with the experiment.

If you have never heard of this experiment before you may now be feeling appalled and thinking that if you had been asked to take part you would have backed out straight away. You would not be alone in presuming this. Before Milgram started the experiment he asked groups of people what they thought they would do if they were put in this situation. Almost everyone said that they would either back out as soon as the experiment started or when they realised that they were delivering painful shocks to the learner. This would seem to be a rational way of responding and would be in line with all our humanistic principles. However, this was not what the results of this experiment showed; 65% of the people who participated in this study went on to the end of the experiment and delivered 450 volts to their innocent learner. Only 35% of subjects were able to resist the authority of the experimenter and refused to continue with the experiment. Milgram then repeated the experiment trying different variations (1965, 1974) to try to find out whether people would be able to resist authority under different conditions. In the first variation he used women as subjects and found that women were just as likely to conform as men. He then moved the experiment to a seedy office in a city suburb (rather than prestigious Yale University); in this venue conformity dropped a little, but still remained quite high. In other variations he put the learner in the same room as the teacher and he also allowed the experimenter to leave the room for brief periods. In the final variation he included two experimenters, each giving conflicting advice to the teacher.

The results of these variations of the original experiment can be seen in *Table 2.1*. What they indicate is that Milgram's original idea is correct. People can easily become involved in a situation where they hurt an innocent third party because they are responding not to innate aggressive tendencies, but to an authority figure who tells them what to do. Obedience drops when the learner is brought into closer proximity to the teacher and it also falls when the experiment was carried out in a less impressive environment. However, even then the number of people who obeyed the experimenter's commands still remained relatively high.

Table 2.1: Results of Milgram's experimental variations (adapted from Pennington, Gillen and Hill, 1999)

Experimental variation	Percentage of subjects giving the maximum shock
Women subjects	65
Less prestigious venue	47.5
Learner in same room	40
Experimenter leaves room	20.5
Conflicting commands	0.0

The most informative results that give us clues about what is actually going on come from the two variations where the experimenter leaves the room and where there are two experimenters giving conflicting advice. In the former, Milgram found that subjects would actually reduce the severity of the shocks when the experimenter left the room, and in the latter when the subjects had 'permission' from one of the experimenters to discontinue the experiment, obedience dropped to 0%. The results of these variations add weight to the argument that the people who participated in these experiments caused pain to an innocent victim because they became locked into a situation from which they could not escape. It was almost as if by agreeing to participate in the experiment the subjects had entered into a contract with the experimenter, a contract which they found very difficult to break even though they were being asked to act in an aggressive way.

When first encountering this experiment of Milgram's the results are so appalling that it may appear that obedience to authority is completely negative. This is not necessarily the case, a certain amount of obedience to authority is essential if society is to function smoothly. We conform to authority in small ways many times a day and we accept that different people have authority in different social situations. For example, while on a train journey we are happy to show our ticket to the ticket collector when he demands to see it; we conform to the authority his role gives him. We would be unlikely to behave in the same way if a fellow passenger demanded to see our ticket because we understand the unwritten social norm that a fellow passenger has no authority to demand this. We would not comply with his request unless he (or she) threatened us in some way or gave some other plausible explanation for seeing the ticket.

In this example, I have argued that you obey the request of the ticket collector to see your ticket because his role gives him the authority to do this. Through socialisation and as members of any given society we understand that it is his job to inspect the tickets of the passengers on the train and he wears a uniform and carries a ticket machine as visual reminders of his position. We accept that he has the authority to ask us to leave the train if we do not have a valid ticket, or report us if we are trying to hitch a free ride. Both the ticket collector and we as passengers know what the role of ticket collector entails and we also understand the limits of this role.

The significance of social roles

Roles are an important part of the explanation of why we obey requests from people in authority. In every society particular roles are invested with authority and other society members are then expected to obey this. This is what happened in Milgram's experiment, the participants obeyed the authority of the white coated experimenter because of the nature of his role and the social context in which the experiment was taking place. Although participants in the experiment felt uncomfortable, they still continued with the experiment because they were told to do so.

How does all this relate to midwifery? Just like the ticket collector the role of midwife gives you the authority to make certain requests of your clients and, like the ticket collector, you may wear a uniform that is a visual signal that indicates the nature of your role. If you ask a woman in labour to lie down so that you can do a vaginal examination (VE), she is likely to comply with your request. It would be quite difficult for her to refuse because within the social context of the hospital she knows that the midwife has the authority to make this request and has the specialised knowledge to know whether a VE is necessary. Although it may be uncomfortable for her to lie down and the VE may be painful she is unlikely to complain and will go along with the demands that are made. Indeed, women who do not comply in this way are likely to be seen as awkward and unhelpful. By refusing to conform they are not fulfilling their role as patient and the delicate balance that is the social microcosm of the labour ward is thrown into disequilibrium.

Another classic experiment that highlights the importance of roles and the influence they have on our behaviour was carried out by Philip Zimbardo (1969). In this experiment student volunteers were asked to take part in a prison simulation exercise. Students were randomly assigned to one of two roles, prisoner or guard. The 'prisoners' were arrested by local police early one Sunday morning and taken to the 'prison' where their clothes were taken away from them. They were then dressed in prison uniform and locked into single cells. The 'guards' were also given uniforms, batons and dark glasses. Both groups, now dressed in appropriate uniforms were left to their own devices but the experiment very quickly got out of hand. The students playing the role of guards became overzealous in their treatment of the prisoners demanding total obedience to their authority. Initially the prisoners reacted to this by refusing to do what the guards told them. The guards responded to this rebellion in more and more punitive ways, making the prisoners clean the toilets with their bare hands and call them 'Mr Correctional Officer'. Eventually, one prisoner refused to eat at all and was put into solitary confine-ment. The other prisoners were told that they could get their colleague out of this situation by giving up one of their blankets but instead of showing solidarity with the rebel, they refused to give up anything to get him out. By now the situation was so bad that the experiment had to be curtailed. Although it had been intended to run the experiment for two weeks, it had to be stopped after only a few days.

It is interesting to reflect on what happened in this experiment and it can be seen that both authority and role had a part to play. Given absolute authority over the 'prisoners' the guards' behaviour towards them became more and more extreme. Although the people playing the role of prisoner knew that this authority was not genuine there was little they could do about it apart from becoming rebellious. The guards responded to this by taking away more and more privileges from the prisoners. The result of this was that eventually the rebellion was not achieving anything and was only serving to take away what little the prisoners had. It was simpler if the prisoners just did what they were told and made life easy for themselves. When one of the prisoners refused to eat the others failed to support him because by now they were only looking after themselves, they were afraid that they would suffer even more losses if they were all punished for the one rebel.

The guards, on the other hand, had been given the task of controlling the prisoners, they were dressed up in their uniforms and there was nothing to stop them behaving just as they liked. Those of you who have taken part in amateur dramatics will appreciate the power of the costume and its ability to change behaviour. In this case, the uniform was an integral part of the role of guard and somehow gave the participants in this experiment the freedom to indulge in behaviour that they would not have dreamed of in normal, everyday life.

Implications for midwifery practice

Although uniforms were originally intended to protect the midwife and mother from disease and midwives are now moving away from wearing them, uniforms in real life invest individuals with power and sometimes alter their behaviour, as with the guards in the prison experiment. Uniforms serve the function of clarifying people's roles and this influences both the wearer of the uniform and the others involved in the situation. Others will have fairly clear ideas what they expect of you as a midwife, and you make assumptions about how you expect the labouring woman to behave. Thus, you are both locked into a situation in which you conform to your roles, in which the midwife has the authority to give the client advice and in which the woman in labour has to do as she is told. In this social microcosm there is a delicate balance of roles and expectations and, just like the prisoners in the experiment described above, a woman in labour may feel that she has a lot to lose if she rebels against the system.

By now I can hear many of you shouting that the scenario that I have just portrayed is unfair and that labour wards are not like this any more. Women in labour are given choices, they are not coerced into doing things that they do not want to do, and they have the freedom to make decisions of their own. Of course this is true, the way women in labour are treated has improved enormously over the past two decades, but the underlying dynamics in the situation are the same even though they may be overlaid with a greater flexibility in approach.

Being aware of the power you have as a professional midwife is essential if you are to improve your practice, and understand the important influence you have on your clients. Women in labour are vulnerable because they are in pain and may feel completely out of control. They are even more susceptible to authority and while it may be convenient to you as a midwife to have a compliant client it is not always in the best interests of the woman. There will be times when your judgement as a professional is essential. You may need to tell a woman what to do; but you have this authority invested in the nature of your professional role, there is no need to use it unless it is imperative that you do so.

Up until now we have looked at social influence in a rather one-sided way in that we have considered how it may affect the woman in labour, but not how the midwife is herself influenced by these social forces. Midwives are subjected to just the same social dynamics as everyone else. For example, a midwife may feel herself to be under great pressure to conform to the common practices of the labour ward in which she is working, when her training and experience indicate that this is not the best way of handling a particular situation. Under these circumstances, an individual may find it very difficult to hold on to her beliefs, and may buckle under the perceived pressure to conform. She may then change her underlying beliefs (private acceptance) or simply go along with the majority until such a time when she is able to express her true opinions again (public compliance).

An experiment by Hofling *et al* (1966) highlighted how the behaviour of nurses could be influenced by obedience to authority with potentially serious consequences for patients. In this study, twenty-two nurses were asked to give an unknown drug (astrogen) to a patient on their ward. This request was made over the telephone by a doctor unfamiliar to them. It was specifically against hospital procedures to administer a drug to a patient without a written request from a doctor. In addition, the doctor requested that the patient be given 20mg of astrogen when the box containing the drug clearly stated that 10mg was the maximum daily dose. Despite this, twenty-one of the twenty-two nurses would have carried out this order if the experiment had not been terminated. Only one subject steadfastly refused to administer the drug to the patient without first seeing the doctor and receiving a written request for the drug. In addition, thirty-three graduate and student nurses were asked to complete a questionnaire in which they said what they thought they would do when confronted with this situation: thirty-one of these subjects stated explicitly that they would politely, but firmly, refuse to carry out the doctor's orders. It would appear from this that behaviour in the real situation is very different from how people thought they would behave when given a hypothetical situation to consider.

Working in a system that is essentially hierarchical the midwife is often subject to the authority of others and she may have to obey rules and dictates passed down from those in positions of power over her. This may not always be easy, particularly if she is told to do something that goes against strongly held beliefs. But, how is it possible to resist these pressures? Up to now, social influence has been described as if it was an inescapable force in society and it has been suggested that all our actions are affected by compliance, conformity and obedience to a greater or lesser extent. While it is true that social influence plays a large part in forming our attitudes and influencing our behaviour, it is obvious that we are not all clones acting in exactly the same way. We see ourselves as unique and our individuality is important to us. It is possible to resist social influence under certain conditions.

Crutchfield (1955) found that conformity was less when subjects were asked to make judgements about matters of taste, rather than objective measurement. He gave participants two pictures to look at. Before the experiment he had shown that one of the pictures was vastly more popular than the other, but he told the subjects that the least popular picture had received more positive ratings. One might have expected that if people were simply conforming they would have chosen the least attractive picture believing it had been rated most highly by others. Crutchfield found that this was not the case, people chose the picture they liked best regardless of the ratings they thought others had given it. It would appear that we are happy to accept variation regarding matters of subjective opinion, but when we believe there is a right answer we do not want to stand out from everyone else. However, if we are confident about the correctness of our opinion this will help us to resist the pressure of the group.

Resisting social influence becomes much easier if we have an ally, just one person who agrees with us and supports our ideas. This chapter began with a description of a meeting in which you were asked to imagine that you were a lone dissenter in a group. Had one other person in the group agreed with you, your feelings of discomfort would have eased considerably and it would have been far easier to express your opinion. In the same way, had you been able to voice your dissenting opinion this would have enabled others to give their views too. Asch (1956) did a variation of his experiment in which just one of the confederates gave the right answer to the line judgement task. This had the effect of allowing the real subject to resist the group pressure and give the right answer too. Even if one accomplice gave a wrong answer that was different to the rest of the group, the subject was able to resist conformity. Under both these conditions conformity in the subjects dropped considerably. Nemeth and Chiles (1988) found that exposing subjects to dissenting minority views also increased resistance to conformity. In this experiment individuals in groups of four were asked to judge the colour of a series of blue stimuli. One of the individuals either consistently or inconsistently judged the stimuli to be 'green'. When subjects were later shown a series of red slides they were able to resist conformity despite the majority view that the slides were 'orange'. The experimenters found that resistance was strengthened regardless of whether subjects had been exposed to consistent or inconsistent dissent. Subjects in a control group with no dissenter did not show such resistance.

The results of these experiments indicate that resisting the majority view can be facilitated if the expression of competing views is encouraged; by speaking your own mind you will give others permission to speak theirs. A false view of consensus can easily be perpetuated when people do not express differing views.

Minority groups can also have a powerful influence and overturn the majority view. Those minority groups with high status and power have the most chance of being able to achieve this, but individuals who have a particular behavioural style or charisma may also be effective (Moscovici, 1985). Einstein and Freud are two examples of people whose ideas were radically different from accepted beliefs but who managed to turn the tide of opinion in their favour. It has been suggested that the behavioural style of these charismatic individuals has four main components:

1. They are consistent in their opinions.
2. They are confident that the ideas they are putting forward are correct.
3. They appear to be objective and unbiased about their ideas.
4. They resist social pressure and abuse (Pennington, Gillen and Hill, 1999).

In addition to these personal qualities, the time at which the dissident ideas appear is crucial. The suffragettes were successful in promoting the cause of universal suffrage for women partly because of their own efforts and partly because the time was ripe for such a change and their arguments for votes for women appeared morally correct.

The issue of responsibility is also important. In the experiments carried out by Milgram, participants constantly asked whether they were responsible for the effects of the electric shocks on the learner. Once the experimenter had reassured them that they were not responsible for the outcome, participants continued with the experiment. Similarly, in a real-life situation, thinking that you will not be held responsible if you are told to do something that goes against your beliefs enables you to continue, even though you may have reservations about what you are doing. Reminding yourself that you are responsible for your actions can be an effective way of helping you to resist authority.

Finally, obedience to authority can be reduced if the authority figure's expertise and motives are queried. In other words, having a healthy disrespect for those in authority will help you to resist the tendency to do as you are told, without first thinking whether you agree with what you are being told to do.

Conclusion

It is important to recognise that conformity can be both a benevolent and malevolent force in society. Conformity is important because it can be seen as the 'glue' that binds society together. If everyone decided to ignore social norms then society as we know it would simply collapse and we would have anarchy. We rely on our human tendency to follow the group and conform to the rules imposed on us by those groups to keep society stable. However, conformity has its dark side too, and this becomes particularly clear when we conform in unthinking ways to adverse group pressure or authority. Under these circumstances, conformity can cause people to act in cruel and inappropriate ways towards others.

It is always a good thing to question and challenge rules that have been imposed on us by those in authority and not simply conform to what is expected. As a group, midwives have generally been pro-active in this and have had a major influence upon changing the conditions in which women give birth. Midwives have instigated and supported changes in practice, such as the routine administration of enemas and supporting women who wish to have home-births. Hopefully, the explanations of social influence provided in this chapter have given you some insight into the mechanisms by which social influence affects behaviour and this knowledge may help you in future to have the courage to resist the tendency to conform.

References

Asch SE (1951) Effects of group pressure upon the modification and distortion of judgement. In: Guetzkow MH, ed. *Groups, Leadership and Men*. Carnegie, Pittsburgh: 177–90

Baron RA, Byrne D (1996) *Social Psychology: Understanding human interaction*. 8th edn. Allyn & Bacon, Boston

Cialdini RB (1995) Principles and techniques of social influence. In: Tesser A, ed. *Advanced Social Psychology*. McGraw Hill, New York

Cialdini RB, Vincent JE, Lewis SK, Catalan J, Wheeler D, Darby BL (1975) Reciprocal concessions procedure for inducing compliance: The door-in-the-face technique. *J Pers Soc Psychol* **31**: 206–15

Cialdini RB, Ascani K (1976) Test of concession procedure for inducing verbal, behavioural and further compliance with a request to give blood. *J Appl Psychol* **61**: 295–600

Crutchfield LH (1955) Conformity and character. *Am Psychol* **10**: 191–8

Freedman JL, Fraser SC (1966) Compliance without pressure: the foot-in-the-door technique. *J Per Soc Psychol* **4**: 195–203

Hofling CK, Brotzman E, Dalrymple S, Graves N, Pierce CM (1966) An experimental study in nurse-physician relationships. *J Nerv Ment Dis* **143**(2): 171–80

Milgram S (1963) Behavioural study of obedience. *J Abnorm Soc Psychol* **67**: 371–8

Milgram S (1965) Some conditions of obedience and disobedience to authority. *Hum Relations* **18**: 57–76

Milgram S (1976) *Obedience to authority: an experimental view.* Harper and Row, New York

Moscovici S (1985) Social Influence and Conformity. In: Lindzey G, Aronson E, eds. *Handbook of Social Psychology.* Random House, New York

Nemeth C, Chiles C (1988) Modelling courage: The role of dissent in fostering independance. *Eur J Soc Psychol* **18**: 275–80

Pennington D, Gillen K, Hill P (1999) *Social Psychology.* Arnold, London

Van Avermaet E (1996) Social influence in small groups. In: Hewstone M, Stroebe MW, Stephenson GM, eds. *Introduction to Social Psychology.* 2nd edn. Blackwell, Oxford: 487–529

Zimbardo P (1969) The human choice: Individuation, reason and order versus deindividuation, impulse and chaos. In: Arnold WJ, Levine D, eds. *Nebraska Symposium on Motivation.* University of Nebraska Press, Lincoln

3

Prejudice and stereotyping or — all Welshmen sing, don't they?

When I teach the topic of prejudice and stereotyping to a group for the first time I usually ask the class to take part in an exercise that they do not always enjoy. I ask them to identify those groups of people in society towards whom they feel an irrational dislike. You may feel that you hold no prejudices, but this is unlikely. Most of us feel mild dislike towards other groups and as a health professional it is particularly important to be aware of your prejudices. For example, Pingitore *et al* (1994) found that many people harbour prejudice towards individuals who are overweight and Maroney and Golub (1992) noted that nurses reported feeling less empathy towards patients who were overweight and were consequently more reluctant to care for them. Any prejudices that you hold, however mild, will have implications for the women you care for.

You might like to try this exercise for yourself. Take a piece of paper and list three groups of people that you feel negatively about. It does not necessarily have to be from a healthcare setting but it will help you to get the most out of this chapter if you do choose groups from those people that you work with. Once you have your list, try to think why it is that you dislike these groups and list your reasons; try to be as honest as you can. Do you have much contact with any individuals from the groups that you have listed?

Most people do not feel comfortable about admitting to these negative feelings about others, they also do not like confronting the fact that their prejudices are largely irrational, often based on very weak evidence. For example, they may have had almost no contact with individuals from the disliked group and suddenly realise that their prejudices are based on hearsay, views expressed in the media and the unconscious internalisation of their parents' prejudiced attitudes.

The exercise does not end here: the next stage is for people to identify times when they have felt themselves to be the victim of prejudice. Some people are lucky and have never been on the receiving end of prejudiced attitudes but it always surprises me how many people have felt themselves, at some point during their lives, to be the victim of prejudice. Perhaps they have been singled out at school because they didn't quite 'fit in', fat children, children who wear glasses and children who are big for their age are often victimised. Students from ethnic minorities frequently report that they have felt discriminated against because of their colour and culture and women also describe instances when they have been affected by prejudiced attitudes.

The important point to note is that almost all of us have prejudices and we all share the tendency to stereotype people into categories. Sometimes these prejudices are very strong and lead to extreme behaviour towards the prejudiced group. The violence directed towards minority groups in contemporary Britain is an example of this. More often, prejudice is much weaker and simply leads the individual to avoid the disliked group and have negative feelings towards the members of that group, but be in no doubt that prejudice exists in all societies in the world and among all classes of people within those societies.

In his book *The Social Animal*, Aronson defines prejudice as:

> *A hostile or negative attitude towards a distinguishable group based on generalizations derived from faulty or incomplete information.*

(Aronson, 1998, p. 299)

This definition encompasses all the features that distinguish prejudice and make it such an insidious force in society. Let us unpack Aronson's definition a little. There are three important ideas contained within it, namely: that prejudice is a hostile or negative attitude, that it is focused towards a distinguishable group and that it springs from faulty or incomplete information about that group. Let us consider each of these concepts more carefully.

A hostile or negative attitude

Although prejudice can be either positive or negative (it is possible to be biased *in favour of* a group), most of us regard prejudice as a negative aspect of human behaviour; indeed, there is little doubt that over the centuries negative prejudice has caused untold human suffering. Atrocities such as the Holocaust of World War II could be said to have sprung directly from prejudiced attitudes towards minority groups. Sexism, racism and ageism are all examples of prejudiced attitudes which act to stereotype individuals and depersonalise them.

Prejudice is focused on a distinguishable group

Prejudice can occur when we falsely assume that all the members of a particular group share the same characteristics. We are all familiar with these generalisations, some relatively harmless examples are: all black people have a good sense of rhythm, all Welsh people can sing, the English are not good at expressing their emotions. While there may be some element of truth in these stereotypes, if you are a member of one of these groups you will know that it is ridiculous to assume that all members of the group share the same characteristics. As an individual you will value the unique characteristics that make you different from anyone else. Nevertheless, although we understand this at a personal level we all continue to maintain stereotypical views of others.

Prejudice is based on faulty or incomplete information

Our prejudices about other groups of people are usually founded on flimsy evidence. Look back at your list of 'disliked' groups; how much do you know about people from those groups? We may not even know individuals who belong to the groups we feel prejudiced against. Indeed, we may actively avoid contact with these groups and then it is easy for prejudices to become entrenched. We may even avoid situations where our established opinions about a group would be challenged.

Why is it important to understand prejudice?

The most obvious answer to this question is that the behavioural manifestations of prejudice have caused enormous amounts of human suffering over the centuries. In all societies people have been victimised and persecuted simply because they have had the misfortune to belong to the 'wrong' group. Jews, gypsies, women, people of colour and the disabled have all been targeted at different times, and countless other groups in different countries throughout the world have experienced the negative consequences of prejudice. This is not a historical phenomenon. The recent wars in Bosnia and Kosova have vividly highlighted how prejudice can create appalling situations where innocent people are murdered, tortured and raped for no other reason than their membership of a particular group.

At the individual level, there is strong evidence to suggest that those who are at the receiving end of prejudice suffer psychologically. In particular, those who experience prejudice suffer from low self-esteem. This is graphically demonstrated in a study that was carried out in a small town in the USA; the results are well recorded in a documentary television programme called *A Class Divided*. A school teacher was so appalled at the assassination of Martin Luther King that she decided to engage her class of nine-year-olds in a learning exercise that would demonstrate to them the devastating effects of prejudice. Her idea was simple, for one day half the class would become members of an 'inferior' group and half would become members of a 'superior group'. Group membership was decided on eye colour.

At the beginning of school one morning the children were told that people with blue eyes were better than those with brown eyes. Blue-eyed people were more intelligent, kinder and generally superior to those who had brown eyes. In recognition of this, brown-eyed children in the classroom had to wear collars around their necks as a visible demonstration of their lower status. Children with brown eyes had to ask to use the drinking fountain, had less time for break and had to wait for the blue-eyed children to finish eating their lunch before they were allowed to eat theirs. During the day the teacher demonstrated in many small ways the superiority of the blue-eyed children over those with brown eyes. The effects of this on the children were enormous. The brown-eyed children became withdrawn and silent, they did not answer questions as readily and achieved less well on tests carried out in the classroom during the day. The blue-eyed children became arrogant and unpleasant. They jeered 'brown eyes' at the others and fights broke out between the two groups.

The next day the roles were reversed. Now the brown-eyed children became the superior group and the blue-eyed children were cast into the role of underdog. On the third and final day of the study the children were debriefed and participated in a lengthy discussion of prejudice and how it felt to be the victim of prejudice. The actions of one child seemed to sum up the whole experience. At the end of the study the children were told that they could remove the collars that they had worn when they were members of the inferior group. This particular boy stood at the waste paper bin and tore his collar into tiny pieces until there was really nothing of it left.

This study demonstrates a number of things about prejudice that are very relevant. Firstly, it has a major impact on those who are its victims. Studies have shown that children of low status groups have their confidence undermined and self-esteem is gradually eroded. This has an impact on their school performance, with low status groups achieving less well in tests than high status groups (Jemmott and Gonzalez, 1989). Secondly, the markers or characteristics that we use to single out those against whom we feel prejudice are entirely arbitrary. In this study it was eye colour. In the study by Jemmott and Gonzalez children were given labels that either said 'boss' or 'helper'. It seems ridiculous to think that eye colour or a label makes any difference to a person. We know that people with blue eyes are not more intelligent than people with brown eyes. In the real world, however, it is different. Skin colour, sex, religious affiliation or any one of a number of features are singled out and used as markers that demonstrate the inferiority of an individual. What can you understand about any individual by focusing on just one of the characteristics that make up their entire personality?

Prejudice against women

Back in 1968, Goldberg carried out a study in which she asked her subjects to evaluate an academic article; half believed that it was written by a woman and half believed that it was written by a man. She found that the article was devalued when it was thought to have been written by a woman and this was true regardless of whether the subject of the article was a 'masculine' field (law and city planning) or a 'feminine' field (dietetics and primary education). Although Goldberg's findings have been supported by several studies, further experiments reveal a more complex picture of this discrimination against women. Ward (1981) replicated Goldberg's study and found:

> *Academic articles attributed to female authors were not rated significantly differently from those attributed to males. Male students, however, devalued female authors per se in status and competence*

(p. 170)

In an experiment carried out with a group of university students and a group of art college students, Colleen Ward (1979) asked subjects to evaluate two paintings: painting A an unnamed water colour and painting B titled 'Girl in Blue'. Her results showed that painting A, which was felt to be of poorer quality than painting B was preferred when it was attributed to a female artist. She also found that the art students who had a certain level of competence in evaluating paintings devalued women artists more than the university students. These results indicate that there is not an overall denigration of women, but that the processes at work are subtler. It is fine to evaluate a woman's work highly when it is regarded as being of poor quality (painting A) or if you do not have expertise in the field. If you regard yourself as competent in a field then you are more likely to denigrate women than if you are a novice. Unfortunately, this tendency has been found to be true of women as well as men and has come to be known as the 'Queen Bee' syndrome (Staines *et al*, 1974).

Ward's experiment was carried out some time ago and it is interesting to consider whether things have changed in the intervening years. After all, feminism has been around that much longer and women are now participating more and more in professional life. It would be encouraging to think that such discrimination was a thing of the past. I suspect that it is still alive and well although in far more subtle forms that are not overt to the observer. This has certainly been found to be the case with racism. As the awareness grew that racism was not socially acceptable, outwardly racist remarks became gradually more toned down and indirect so that now, although blatant discrimination and gross stereotypes are rejected, reasons that are seemingly non-racial are given as justifications for opposing racial change (Pettigrew, 1989). The existence of groups such as the British National Party in Britain and their equivalents in France and Germany demonstrate that racism, albeit in these more elusive forms, is far from dead.

A note about prejudice and stereotyping

Both prejudice and stereotyping are examples of what might be described as a universal human tendency to group and classify information in order to make sense of it. While this does not condone prejudice, it does help us to understand why it happens.

Everyday of our lives, from the moment we are born, we are confronted with a bewildering amount of material to process. Our senses are constantly bombarded with information about the physical world, the social world and our own internal world. In order to make this huge amount of information more manageable, we categorise it, put it into pigeon-holes and link together things that we perceive to be similar. We use both our perceptions and what we have learned about the world during our lifetime to do this. This process makes the information easier to handle. It would be almost impossible to perceive everything we encounter as a completely new experience, we simply would not be able to cope with the quantity of information, neither would we be able to make meaning from these perceptions.

To get a sense of the usefulness of our ability to group and categorise information try the following exercise; you will need a pencil and paper to do it, and it's more fun if you can get a friend to help you. Below are two lists each containing twenty-five words. If you are doing the exercise by yourself, read through the first list fairly slowly reading from left to right. Make sure that you read each word once only and do not attempt to memorise the list. If you are doing the exercise with someone else, ask them to read out the list to you. As soon as you have finished reading the list (or your partner has finished reading the list to you) take your piece of paper and write down as many words as you can remember. When you reach a point where you cannot remember any more words, stop and count up the number of words that you have recalled.

Cat	Sheet	Run	Sugar	Lorry
Blanket	Jump	Car	Saucer	Rabbit
Milk	Hop	Duvet	Mouse	Bus
Pillow	Van	Leap	Teapot	Dog
Cup	Hampster	Mattress	Train	Swim

Figure 3.1: Memory task — list one

Now repeat the exercise in exactly the same way with the second list of words. Make sure that you read the words from left to write, line by line from top to bottom.

Candle	Match	Wick	Wax	Burn
Cow	Sheep	Pig	Horse	Goat
Book	Paper	Pen	Crayon	Pencil
Table	Chair	Sofa	Stool	Cushion
Grin	Happy	Laugh	Smile	Chuckle

Figure 3.2: Memory task — list two

I would predict that you managed to remember more of the second list than of the first list and the reason that you did this was because the words in the second list had been grouped into categories. The task of remembering more words was simplified because you could think of each category and then link words within that category together. It seems to be a natural tendency in humans to find patterns in everything they perceive whether it is visual information, language, or the characteristics of a friend and then, in order to make sense of these patterns we classify them into groups and label them under a category heading.

It might help to illustrate this with another example. Consider the word 'dog' and try to imagine an example of a dog. Now try to think what are the features that make a dog a dog and not a cat? Although dogs vary enormously in size and shape we recognise dogs as dogs when we see them in the street and we understand that all dogs share particular features and characteristics. We know that dogs are part of a larger group called mammals and we are able to recognise how dogs may be similar to and/or different from other mammals (cats and hamsters, for example). We also know that there are many different breeds of dog who share these features of 'dogginess' but who also have characteristics that arc individual to that particular breed. We are able to categorise dogs as mammals and poodles as dogs by using the information that we have acquired over the years. Some of this information will be based on characteristics for which we have evidence, eg. all dogs bark. But some of our ideas about dogs may be based on less concrete information, for example, having listened to the news over the past few years we may believe that all pit bull terriers are dangerous and should be put down. Categorising all pit bull terriers in this negative way is an example of prejudice; no doubt there are pit bull terriers that are not dangerous. In fact, the dangerous ones may even be in the minority.

When we classify our world in this way we are simplifying the amount of information that we have to process. Most of the time our ability to do this serves us well, indeed, we encourage this skill in our children by giving them exercises in which they practice it. For example, sorting and classifying objects which share certain characteristics. However, when we classify groups of people in this way and attach a negative evaluation to particular characteristics then that is prejudice and this leads to many problems in society.

> *A network of intergroup categorizations is omnipresent in the social environment; it enters into our socialization and*

> *education all the way from 'teams' and 'team spirit' in the*
> *primary and secondary education through teenage*
> *groupings of all kinds to social, national, racial, ethnic,*
> *religious or age groups.*

(Tajfel, Flament, Billig and Bundy, 1971, p. 153)

We have seen that the tendency to categorise information leads to stereotyping and prejudice and also that prejudice exists in all societies — but what causes prejudice? What marks prejudice out from stereotyping is the negative evaluation attached to it, how does this arise? Social psychologists have offered a number of explanations that attempt to answer this question, they fall roughly into two categories; those that look for reasons for prejudice within the individual and those that explain prejudice through group processes.

Causes of prejudice: explanations based on the individual

Displaced aggression or 'scapegoating'

We are probably all familiar with the experience of taking out our frustration on some inanimate object or powerless creature. This tends to happen when we cannot vent our feelings on the real source of our frustration, perhaps because the frustrating entity is more powerful than ourselves or because it is something vague and non-specific and therefore impossible to attack. When we find that colleagues in work have gone over our heads about an important decision or the insurance company spends months sorting out an insurance claim, we may well come home and kick the cat or be verbally aggressive to members of our family. These victims of our anger are not the real source of our frustration but are 'scapegoats' taking the brunt of frustrations that cannot be expressed elsewhere.

Aronson (1998) points out that the idea of a scapegoat comes from biblical times when a real goat would be used symbolically to carry into the wilderness all the anger and frustrations of a group of people. Nowadays, social psychologists suggest that groups in society may be made into scapegoats and are labelled with all the difficulties and problems that other people cannot escape from and have no control over. People from ethnic minorities are blamed because there is high unemployment and they are accused of taking all the jobs that could go to the indigenous population. Young blacks are blamed for the rise in crime. This scapegoating eventually leads to prejudice and groups are assumed to epitomise all the negative qualities that other people's attitudes have invested them with.

In addition, we are not comfortable with the idea of directing aggression at a group for no good reason, we tend to justify our hostile attitudes and acts of aggression by dehumanising that group. It is much easier to be negative towards those who you feel to be unworthy, than towards people whom you believe to be your equal.

Prejudice through conformity

It has been suggested that we may be prejudiced simply because we are conforming to the mores of the society in which we live. If we grow up in a situation in which prejudiced attitudes are the norm then it may be difficult to see the world in any other way. This may continue until we are exposed to different ideas through education, the media or through involvement with the groups against whom we are prejudiced. This cause of prejudice is largely borne of ignorance and irrational fear of groups that are 'different' to our own familiar groups.

Prejudice and self-esteem

We have already seen that prejudice causes low self-esteem but there is a large body of evidence that indicates that those low in self-esteem tend to be more prejudiced themselves. Crocker *et al* (1987) demonstrated this in a study of college students where those low in self-esteem were generally more negative about others than students with higher levels of self-esteem. Such a finding highlights why prejudice is so difficult to eradicate in society: prejudice not only causes low self-esteem in those who are its victims, but is in turn generated by low self-esteem.

The prejudiced personality

Adorno *et al* (1950) suggested that the cause of prejudice was rooted within the psyche of the individual. In other words, certain people were more prone to become prejudiced than others. Using a Freudian perspective it was argued that a prejudiced personality type could be measured by means of a simple personality test, the F-scale (F stood for fascist). Individuals who had this personality type shared certain things in common, such as authoritarian parents and a history of severe physical punishment in childhood. As adults, prejudiced personalities manifested as a tendency to be extremely deferential to those in authority over them, but overbearing towards those weaker than themselves. This became known as the authoritarian personality and was characterised by racist or fascist tendencies and dogmatic, reactionary opinions.

While it is tempting to believe that some people are more prone to exhibit prejudice because of their personality, Adorno's research has been heavily censured. The F-scale itself was criticised because of the way it was constructed, the questionnaire items are all worded in such a way that agreement with the statements represents the presence of the prejudiced attitude (Brown, 1965). Questionnaires should contain both positive and negative statements to prevent respondents falling into response sets (ie. simply agreeing with statements all the time). It was argued that the results obtained from the test were more to do with acquiescence on the part of the subjects than authoritarianism (Cohn, 1953). When Bass (1955) reversed the items of the F-scale so that disagreement with them indicated authoritarianism, several participants agreed with both the positive and negative form of the statement.

The work was also criticised because the sample used was not representative of a normal population. All the participants were members of at least one formal organisation and were in fact recruited to the study through these organisations, perhaps such people are not typical? There are many more criticisms of Adorno's study which a not appropriate to go into here (see Brown, 1965), but quite apart from the methodological problems, this approach does not explain social aspects of prejudice that have been observed. For example, why is prejudice more prevalent in some cultures than others and in some sub-groups more than others, and why does it tend to fluctuate with time? As Brown asks:

If prejudice is to be explained via individual differences amongst people, how can it then be manifested in a whole population?

(1996, p. 533)

In the histories of most nations there have been times when prejudice is more obvious than at other times. Until recently in South Africa prejudice in the form of apartheid was actually sanctioned and legalised by the state, in Europe and North America prejudice against women was active during the witch hunts from the fourteenth to the seventeenth century (Ussher, 1991).

It would appear that individualistic explanations of prejudice are not sufficient to demonstrate its various manifestations in society. There seem to be forces at work that are dependent upon individuals' membership of groups, we therefore need to look at how group membership influences prejudice.

Group identity and prejudice

Chapter 2 discussed the significance of group membership to most of us; few people choose to live alone and the vast majority of individuals actively seek to belong to groups. We tend to identify with particular groups and see ourselves as similar to other group members. Belonging to groups helps us to define ourselves and feel part of society. Identification with a particular group leads to the formation of what psychologists call in-groups and out-groups. In-groups are those groups to which we have membership and access and they are the groups with which we identify ourselves. There is a tendency to make assumptions about and categorise the characteristics of the members of in-groups and out-groups. We see in-group members as 'like-us' and their characteristics as positive and we see out-group members as 'diffcrent-from-us' and negative. Although this way of looking at things makes us feel good about ourselves and the groups to which we belong, it also allows us to develop prejudiced attitudes towards members of the out-group.

Status and power needs

As we have seen, we judge our standing in society by comparison with others and nobody wants to feel that they have no status or are powerless. It helps us to feel better about ourselves if we feel that we belong to a group that is more powerful than another group. If you are a person who has a reasonable standing in society then this is probably not a problem for you, you are reasonably secure in your status. However, if you belong to a group that comes low down on the socioeconomic ladder then one could predict that as a member of this group you will need someone to feel superior to (Wills, 1981).

As Aronson (1998) suggests:

*An individual who is low on the socioeconomic hierarchy may need the pressure of a downtrodden minority group in order to be able to feel superior to **somebody**.*

(p. 323, author's emphasis)

Crocker *et al* (1987) found evidence to support this view. Working with students, she found that women who were members of low status college groups expressed more prejudice than those in higher status groups. Research by Dollard (1987) also found that low-status white people are more likely to be prejudiced against blacks than high status whites.

It is difficult to know from these studies whether we can argue that there is a human need for status and power. Other explanations for these findings are possible, for example, people of lower socio-economic status could be generally less well educated than those of higher status, therefore their prejudice could stem from ignorance. Another possibility is that people of low socioeconomic status are less secure in terms of their position in society and are more threatened by other groups, prejudice then becomes a way of defending oneself against the perceived threat. This leads us to another cause of prejudice.

Economic and political competition

At most times in any given society there are not enough resources to go around the entire population. This leads to inequalities between groups with some people owning the large majority of the wealth and most of the power. Competition for economic and political resources can create a situation where groups set themselves up against each other. Racial, ideological and religious differences can then exacerbate the tension, with the in-group competing against the out-group for scarce resources and making all kinds of negative assumptions about the out-group which eventually lead to prejudiced attitudes.

The relationship between competition and prejudice has been shown in several studies. Dollard (1987) described how in a small town in the USA prejudice against German immigrants increased when jobs became scarce. A similar pattern emerged with Chinese immigrants in the USA in the nineteenth century. Initially, when the Chinese were trying to mine gold in California they were demonised and described as, 'depraved and vicious... gross gluttons... blood-thirsty and inhuman' (Roberts, quoted in Aronson, 1995, p. 325).

Later, when doing hard and unpleasant work on the railroad, they were described as hard-working and honest. Opinions about them changed yet again when the Civil War ended and there was once again strong competition for a limited number of jobs.

The situation that currently exists in Northern Ireland is a good example of how political and economic competition can lead to prejudice, which eventually escalates into violence between groups. There are ideological and religious differences between the two warring factions. There is competition for land: the Catholics believe that they are the indigenous population and Northern Ireland belongs to them, and there is competition for limited resources. Economically the Catholics in Northern Ireland tend to be poorer and feel discriminated against in terms of jobs and education. The situation is unlikely to be resolved unless the sources of the competition are removed and despite recent peace initiatives this seems unlikely in the foreseeable future.

World-wide, we see many more examples of similar situations; the war in former Yugoslavia could largely be explained through economic and political competition leading to hatred between the Bosnians and the Serbs. The struggle between the Israelis and Palestinians is about land, power and the attempts of one group of people to dominate the other. In a hospital setting, prejudice between groups can be related to competition over expertise within a particular area.

Is it inevitable then that political and economic competition will lead to prejudice? A well-known experiment by Sherif *et al* (1961) demonstrated both how prejudice could be created between two groups, and how it could be broken down again if conditions were manipulated correctly. Sherif *et al* carried out this experiment in a boy's camp in the USA. The boys were around twelve years of age and were all psychologically well-adjusted. At the beginning of the experiment none of the boys knew each other, but after a few days they were divided into two groups called the Eagles and the Rattlers. Intergroup conflict between the two groups was set up by encouraging the boys to identify strongly with their group and by artificially manipulating a series of situations in which one group lost out to the other. For example, both groups were invited to a picnic tea, but one group was asked fifteen minutes earlier than the other. By the time the second group arrived much of the best food was gone. The two groups were encouraged to compete against each other in games such as tug-of-war. The winning group in these games received a cup and each member of the group a brand-new penknife. Members of the other group received nothing at all. In a short space of time the two groups who previously had existed peacefully together were actively hostile towards each other. There were no intergroup friend-ships (even though these had existed before the start of the experiment) and there was occasional violence. Individuals identified strongly with their own group and rejected and jeered at individuals belonging to the out-group.

In order to reduce the conflict and prevent all-out war, Sherif and his co-workers had to set up a number of situations in which the two groups needed to cooperate in order to achieve an outcome that was mutually beneficial to both groups. Sherif called these super-ordinate goals. For example, the truck carrying the boys back to camp after a trip 'broke down'. It was obviously in the interest of both groups to get the truck working again otherwise a long walk back to camp was inevitable. The groups had to pool their resources in order to achieve the desired end. After a number of similar events conflict between the two groups was reduced and the hostility that had so easily been generated was gradually broken down.

Prejudice by virtue of group membership

The results of Sherif's experiment imply that prejudice can be created almost arbitrarily simply by group membership. The Eagles and Rattlers were created purely for the purposes of an experiment, the children who participated had no prior allegiance to either of these groups. Tajfel *et al* (1971) have done a number of studies on minimal groups, that is groups formed specifically for experimental purposes with no prior affiliation, and have found evidence to suggest that simply knowing that you belong to a group is sufficient to generate intergroup bias.

> *... there are insistent indications that competition is not a necessary condition for creating discrimination between the in-group and the out-group.*
>
> (Tajfel *et al*, 1971, p. 151)

In a simple experiment in which groups of fourteen- and fifteen-year-old boys were divided into groups based on their performance on a perceptual task, it was found that participants were more likely to reward members of their own group than members of the other group. Tajfel *et al* interpret their results in terms of what they call a 'built-in' social norm to form social groups, even when individual members gain little or no personal profit from doing so.

Prejudice and the midwife: implications for midwifery practice

Imagine that you are assisting a woman in labour who belongs to a group about which you feel a mild degree of prejudice. I mentioned earlier in this chapter that I usually ask midwives who I am teaching to identify groups that they feel prejudiced against. Groups that come up frequently are: women who are overweight, members of the National Childbirth Trust (NCT) and women with very detailed and rigid birth plans. Your prejudice about these categories of people will mean that you will interpret this individual woman and what she does during labour through the lens of your negative attitude and this will subtly influence your behaviour towards her. Your professional skills and training should prevent your behaviour from being overtly negative but in small ways it is likely that your prejudice will demonstrate itself. Perhaps this will be manifested in the way that you talk to the client or the way that you touch her. Maybe you will be less tolerant of behaviour that you would have accepted in someone else or you interpret behaviour as an example of 'that kind of person' without looking beneath the surface for other possible causes. For example, someone with a minutely detailed birth plan may be exceptionally anxious about labour and birth and this is her way of coping with and controlling that anxiety. The danger is that our prejudices prevent us from seeing each individual as unique; they act as blinkers that hinder us from looking for wider intrapersonal and individual explanations of people's reactions to events.

Of course, prejudice is not one-sided, it is not only the midwife who may have negative attitudes towards particular groups. Labouring women come to antenatal classes and onto the labour ward with prejudices of their own and you will have to be aware of and cope with the behaviour this creates. Similarly, prejudices often exist between groups of health professionals and this can lead to tension in the work place.

Earlier in the chapter we saw how group membership alone can create negative attitudes towards the out-group. Such negative evaluations can be created very easily in minimal groups and it follows that prejudice based on social categorisation is liable to arise in any work place. It seems to me that it is probably more likely to happen in settings where there is a well-defined hierarchy and where several well-defined groups are engaged in similar tasks. Hospitals meet both these criteria and we might expect to find prejudiced attitudes existing between groups of healthcare workers.

This might be particularly rife in the case of midwife/

obstetrician relationships where a degree of competition might exist regarding expertise, and where both groups may have quite different views about how to deal with women in labour. All-out war is probably averted because midwives and obstetricians are professionals and would not allow personal feelings to get in the way of their duties and also share superordinate goals, ie. the safe delivery of a healthy baby and the well being of the mother. But, such negative attitudes lurking just below the surface can lead to tensions and an unpleasant working environment.

Conclusion

It should be apparent to the reader by now that prejudice exists throughout all societies and in all individuals to a greater or lesser extent. If we are honest with ourselves we will probably accept that there are some groups in society to whom we have a hostile attitude and who we stereotype in negative ways. In the caring professions, developing an awareness of one's prejudices is particularly important as these can influence behaviour, which in turn may have a profound effect on the clients. A midwife's attitude towards a woman in labour could have a major impact on her experience of childbirth.

Although there are very large intrapersonal variations in the strength of individual prejudices, some people allow their prejudices to influence their behaviour towards the out-group more than others. Being aware of your prejudices can help you to modify your behaviour and mitigate its effects, although this alone may not eradicate them.

In summary, the interpersonal nature of prejudice prevents us from dealing with people at an intrapersonal level. Because we have the tendency to categorise information, we can easily forget that the person we are dealing with is an individual and make assumptions about group characteristics. In doing this, it is very easy to forget that each woman in labour comes onto the ward with her own unique set of personal circumstances, which will influence how she reacts to and copes with the process of giving birth. Although her membership of any particular cultural group is relevant and will influence how she copes with labour, she remains an individual and should be responded to as such.

References

Adorno TW, Frenkel-Brunswick E, Levinson DJ, Sanford RN (1950) *The Authoritarian Personality*. Harper, New York

Aronson E (1995) *The Social Animal*. 7th edn. WH Freeman, New York

Aronson E (1998) *The Social Animal*. 8th edn. WH Freeman, New York

Bass BM (1955) Authoritarianism or acquiescence? *J Abnorm Soc Psychol* **51**: 616–23

Brown R (1965) *Social Psychology*. Free Press, New York

Brown R (1996) Intergroup Relations. In: Hewstone M, Stroebe W, Stephenson GM, eds. *Introduction to Social Psychology*. Blackwell, Oxford: 530–61

Cohn TS (1953) The relation of the F-scale to a response to answer positively. *Am Psychologist* **8**: 385

Crocker J, Thompson LL, McGraw KM, Ingerman C (1987) Downward comparison, prejudice and evaluations of others: effects of self-esteem and threat. *J Pers Soc Psychol* **52**: 907–16

Dollard J (1987) *Class and Caste in a Southern Town*. Yale University Press, New Haven

Goldberg P (1968) Are women prejudiced against women? *Transaction* **5**: 28–32

Jemmott JB, Gonzalez E (1989) Social status, the status distribution and performance in small groups. *J Appl Soc Psychol* **19**(7): 584–98

Maroney D, Golub S (1992) Nurses' attitudes toward obese persons and certain ethnic groups. *Percept Mot Skills* **75**: 387–91

Pettigrew TF (1989) The nature of modern racism in the united States. *Rev Int Psychol Soc* **2**(3): 291–303

Pingitore R, Dugooni BL, Tindale RS, Spring B (1994) Bias against overweight job applicants in a simulated employment interview. *J Appl Psychol* **79**: 909–17

Sherif M, Harvey OJ, White BJ, Hood WR, Sherif CW (1961) *Intergroup Conflict and Cooperation: the robbers cave experiment*. University of Oklahoma, Norman, OK

Staines G, Jayaratne J, Tavris C (1974) The Queen Bee syndrome. *Psychol Today* **7**(8): 55–60

Tajfel H, Flament C, Billig MG, Bundy RP (1971) Social categorization and intergroup behaviour. *Eur J Soc Psychol* **1**(2): 149–78

Ussher J (1991) *Women's Madness: misogyny or mental illness?* Harvester Wheatsheaf, Hemel Hempstead

Ward C (1979) Differential evaluation of male and female expertise: Prejudice against women? *Br J Clin Psychol* **18**: 65–9

Ward C (1981) Prejudice against women: who, when and why? *Sex Roles* **7**(2): 163–71

Wills TA (1981) Downward comparison principles in social psychology. *Psychol Bull* **90**: 245–71

4

Perception of ourselves and others: what you think you see is not always what you get

Imagine a situation in which you are meeting a pregnant woman for the first time, it could be in the booking clinic or on the labour ward or even in the delivery room. To do this short exercise it might be helpful to think of an example from real life, perhaps a situation that has occurred recently. Do not worry if you cannot think of an example from a midwifery context, thinking of meeting someone for the first time in any social setting will work just as well. Being as honest as you can, answer the following questions:

- what was the first thing you noticed about this person, what aspects of their appearance, mannerisms and language were salient and helped you to form an impression of them?
- did you make judgements based on the way that they looked, or the way that they spoke?
- were you influenced by the way they were dressed?
- did their accent have an impact on you; were you able to identify them as middle or working class and was this important to you?
- did you think this person would be an 'easy' or 'difficult' patient?

After attempting to answer these questions you might be thinking that none of them are relevant to what happens to you when you meet someone for the first time. Perhaps you are feeling indignant at the suggestion that such processes of classification go on in your mind. It may be that you try to be impartial and avoid making assumptions about a person until you know them better. Possibly you objected to the word 'judgement' believing that you never make judgements about others. In practice, it is unlikely that you formed no impression at all of your new acquaintance, as Asch comments:

> *We look at a person and immediately a certain impression of his character forms itself in us. A glance, a few spoken*

words are sufficient to tell us a story about a highly complex matter.

(1946, p. 533)

The purpose of this chapter is to explore what psychologists have discovered about how we perceive others and what influences us in this. In psychological terminology this is referred to as social cognition.

A note about social cognition

In psychology, the word cognition generally refers to all those mental processes that involve thinking and perception including memory, attention and language, it also encompasses how humans organise the information that enters the brain via the senses. Social cognition refers to these same mental processes but focuses on how they are used to make sense of the social context that surrounds us. It is important to realise that cognition is never a passive process, individuals actively attempt to understand and make sense of what they perceive in the environment and this is also true of social situations. As we have already seen when looking at stereotyping and prejudice, we also try to organise information into manageable chunks that can be understood more easily.

Differences between perceiving objects and perceiving people

The perceptual processes that we use when observing, say a chair, and observing another person are essentially the same — the eyes take in the information from the environment and convey this information to the brain which then interprets and makes sense of the scene before it. However, there are some important differences that are fundamental to understanding how we perceive others. If I were to ask a group of twenty people to describe a particular chair, assuming the lighting conditions were the same for all the people, I could be reasonably sure that each of their descriptions of the chair would be similar. If I asked twenty people to describe one of their colleagues I have no doubt that each of their descriptions would vary considerably. How each individual described their colleague would depend on how well they knew them, whether they liked them, whether they found them attractive and so on. Although the perceptual processes involved are fundamentally the same, the way we make sense of these observations is different when the object of our gaze is another person and not an inanimate object. When observing social situations there is a two-way relationship; we use our cognitive processes to make sense of social situations but we are also influenced by the social context in which we are making our observations.

Part of the reason for this difference is that our interactions (if we may call them this) with inanimate objects are one-sided. I may interact with the chair by sitting on it but the chair does not respond to this. On the other hand, our interactions with others are always just that, interactions with both participants involved in the exchange, interpreting the behaviour of the other, and modifying their behaviour accordingly; the actions of the one influencing the actions of the other in a continuous modifying and altering gavotte of social exchange.

Pennington, Gillen and Hill (1999) argue that there are four fundamental differences in our perception of objects and our perception of people.

1. People are causal agents and attempt to control their world while inanimate objects do not. In other words, the chair cannot do anything to get you to like it, but people can and do try to influence how others see them. The way they talk and dress, what they talk about and how frequently they smile are modified to suit people and situations.
2. We are influenced by others and our conduct changes in response to how they behave towards us. To stay with the example of the chair — however many times we observe it, the chair will always be the same, but people can be pleasant or unpleasant, charming or obnoxious, boring or entertaining and our behaviour towards them will alter accordingly.
3. When we describe other people much of what we say is not directly observable but is inferred from their behaviour, these inferences are not always accurate and are frequently based on incomplete information. Our prejudices also influence our judgements.
4. We are all likely to agree on whether the cover of a chair is black or grey, chintz or plain, but it is almost impossible to determine whether our inferences about other people are accurate or not.

To this list I would add a fifth; our perception of others is more likely to have some emotional involvement. It would be unusual if we felt liking or warmth when we gazed at a chair, but we frequently feel some level of emotion when we observe other people. We may feel warmth, affection, liking, attraction, dislike, revulsion, indifference, in fact, the whole range of emotion from one extreme to another.

All of this adds up to the fact that generally we do not regard other people with whom we interact in emotionally neutral ways. Our observations of others are tied up with feelings that are influenced by a whole range of ideas. Ideas that are grounded in the social context, our personal style, our history and knowledge of human behaviour and our beliefs about what kind of person this might be.

Forming impressions of others

People try to make sense of each other in order to guide their own actions and interactions. Given these concerns, (a) perceivers must be accurate enough for current purposes, (b) they must create informative but workable structures, and (c) the entire process must be highly sensitive to people's goals, sets, motives, and needs.

(Fiske, 1993)

Many people are of the opinion that what you think about someone when you first meet them is highly significant and an accurate reflection of what that person is like. It is often believed that this 'first impression' is a good indicator of how you will get along with someone in the long term. This popular myth is reflected in the notion of 'love at first sight'. While it is difficult to understand what is going on in the psyche of a person who experiences love at first sight, it is unlikely that anyone can have a full understanding of another individual on the basis of a single encounter. Despite this comment, recent research in the field of social cognition suggests that we are able to glean enough information from a first encounter for our purposes. In other words, in terms of social cognitive abilities people are 'good-enough' perceivers (Zebrowitz, 1990).

First impressions are frequently mediated by our individual theories about personality. Stereotypes we may hold about accent, social class, attractiveness, occupation and styles of dress will also affect how we perceive a person. Implicit personality theory is the term psychologists use to describe these idiosyncratic rules of thumb which are based on things that we have been told as children, past experiences, and stereotypes. Whether we are aware of them or not, we all have our own individual personality theories that help us to classify and make judgements about the people we meet. Such individual theories can be helpful in enabling us to make decisions about who we are likely to get on with, who we will like, who we might dislike and so on. However, as a health professional you need to be self-aware, as implicit personality theory can frequently cause you to make inaccurate and wrong assumptions about people. The following anecdote might help to illustrate this.

A hospital consultant that I know told me about a management course in which he had taken part. One exercise involved the participants in making some predictions about other course members. Although the people involved knew nothing about each other, apart from their occupations, they had to say what paper they thought the other person read, what car they drove and which political party they had voted for in the last election. The consultant's partner thought that he would read *The Daily Telegraph*, would drive a BMW and would have voted Conservative. In fact, this particular consultant read *The Times* and *The Guardian*, drove an old Mini and had voted Labour at the last general election. In this case, first impressions had been wildly inaccurate. The consultant's partner in this exercise had used generalisations based on stereotypes, to make many assumptions about aspects of his lifestyle. He had constructed in his own mind a person who did not exist. In a real life situation such assumptions might also have led this individual to think he would not get along with the consultant because of the personal characteristics he had imagined.

In the same way that we can be misled into making judgements about people based on generalisation and stereotypes, Asch (1946) found that we tend to make global assessments of personality and that certain personality traits are extremely influential in this process. Two groups of subjects were given lists of character-qualities identical apart from one adjective. Group A received the list:

❖ intelligent, skilful, industrious, *warm*, determined, practical, cautious.

While group B received the list:

❖ intelligent, skilful, industrious, *cold*, determined, practical, cautious.

The subjects participating in the experiment were then asked to write a brief account of what they thought this imaginary person would be like.

Asch believed that the character-qualities *warm* and *cold* would influence subjects into making assumptions about the existence of other personality traits. Indeed, this hypothesis was borne out by the results of the experiment with a very different picture of the fictitious person emerging from the accounts of the two groups. Subjects in group A who had received the list of adjectives including the word warm, tended to write more positive accounts that suggested that the person would also be generous, wise, happy, good-natured and sociable. Subjects who had been given the adjective trait cold gave low ratings for these traits. However, similar numbers in both groups believed the person would be persistent, serious, strong and honest.

Table 4.1: Summary of Asch's results

Perceived quality	Group A	Group B
Generous	91	8
Wise	65	25
Happy	90	34
Humorous	77	13
Reliable	94	99
Important	88	99
Humane	86	31
Persistent	100	97
Serious	100	99
Strong	98	95
Honest	98	94

In a variation of this experiment Asch found that the impact of the words warm and cold changed when surrounded by different adjectives. To one group he gave the list:

❖ obedient, weak, shallow, *warm*, unambitious, vain.

Another group received the list:

❖ vain, shrewd, unscrupulous, *warm*, shallow, envious.

Yet a third group were given:

❖ intelligent, skilful, sincere, *cold*, conscientious, helpful, modest.

He now found that in the first two cases warmth was no longer regarded as a positive quality but was seen to indicate negative and insincere characteristics. In the third case, coldness now surrounded by positive qualities, was viewed as a superficial trait, indicative of shyness that would quickly disappear once the person was better known.

Asch also found evidence that what we hear first about a person influences us more than what comes later (primacy effect). Although this finding may at first appear unimportant it becomes more serious when extrapolated to a real-life situation such as a court room. Pennington (1982) found evidence to suggest that juries are more influenced in the verdicts by evidence that they hear first, particularly when the court case is long.

Asch's experiments can be criticised on many grounds: being laboratory-based it cannot be said to be representative of real-life situations, which are vastly more complex and involve the dynamic interaction between two or more people. The information on character qualities is oversimplified and bears little resemblance to the information that would normally be available when forming an impression of another person. The descriptions generated by the subjects are in fact artefacts of the experiment, they were only produced because the experimental procedure demanded it. Under normal circumstances impression formation is not such a static process but changes over time. It is a two-way process too; when people interact they alter their behaviour slightly according to the circumstances. Despite these difficulties the findings do allow us to draw out a number of useful points which are relevant to the health professional.

Let us consider a situation that is hypothetical, but may well occur several times in the course of your working day. As we have already seen, in face-to-face situations we have a large amount of material that we can draw on in constructing a view of another but how often do we only have descriptions of clients provided for us by other colleagues? How much does this then colour our opinions and behaviour towards that individual? Asch's experiment gives us some insight into this. It shows how easy it can be to influence someone's perception of an individual, even before that person has had a chance to interact with him or her. This can be particularly true if the form of words chosen link in with another's stereotypes. For example, I know from teaching midwives that there is a popular stereotype about teachers in labour, the midwifery profession generally regards these women as being 'stroppy' and difficult to manage. Just imagine that as she changes shift one midwife comments to another, 'She's a typical teacher'. What does this tell the midwife who is just beginning her shift? How does it influence the situation and does it help? Just because one midwife has found a woman difficult, does not mean that another midwife will interact in the same way.

Asch's experiment illustrates our ability and willingness to imagine an entire personality from very little information. It also demonstrates how one assumed personality trait can affect the entire picture that is built up of a person. In normal face-to-face situations we have a large amount of material that we can draw on in constructing a view of a client, but how often do we only have descriptions provided for us by other colleagues? How much does this then influence our opinions and behaviour towards that individual? Other researchers have noted that negative information about a person is more salient than positive information (Fiske, 1980). It is also true that once a negative impression of a person has been formed it is far more difficult to change (Pennington, Gillen and Hill, 1999). There is a need for caution before describing a client as 'awkward and difficult' to another colleague, even when that has been your honest experience of them.

The experiment highlights the power of language. In this respect, the simplicity of the design is helpful as it strips away all the extraneous information that would normally be available in a real-life setting and forces the subjects to fall back on the meaning of the words used to describe the character qualities. It is clear that the words used both by Asch and his subjects in their accounts are neither emotionally neutral nor value-free. Each adjective reflects personal qualities that have social meanings. The value we attach to these qualities then affects whether the overall description of the imaginary person is positive or negative. We rarely think about the impact that our language may have on others, but the words we use to describe clients could conceivably have far-reaching consequences in terms of how other health professionals respond to them.

Finally, thinking back to *Chapter 2*, the experiment illustrates how easy it is to get large numbers of people to do apparently pointless tasks.

Self-fulfilling prophecies

Before we move on to look at another aspect of social perception it is important to mention the idea of the **self-fulfilling prophecy**. In many ways this can be simply described as, 'you get what you expect to get'. For example, if you expect a woman in labour to be difficult to manage and challenging then she will tend to fulfil those expectations. The self-fulfilling prophecy is illustrated very well in a famous experiment by two researchers called Rosenthal and Jacobsen (1968). These psychologists carried out a piece of research in a primary school classroom. In the first phase of the experiment all of the children were given an intelligence test, which was supposed to pinpoint those children who were about to make sudden gains in intellectual development. In fact, the test used was simply an ordinary intelligence test that measured each child's level of ability. Twenty children in the class were then picked out at random and teachers were told that these were the children who were about to have an intellectual growth spurt. Very quickly teachers began to rate these children as more curious, more interested and happier than other children in the class and when IQ was measured again over a two-year period, children made significantly greater gains than would have been expected by chance.

It is not completely clear how the self-fulfilling prophecy works, but it is probably due to quite subtle social interactions. For example, if you expect a woman to be difficult, then perhaps you are less friendly and warm in your interactions with her, possibly your voice inflection reflects this or maybe you do not seem terribly interested in what the mother says when she tries to communicate with you. The mother sensing this becomes a little wary, she may feel angry and anxious and begin to complain more, which confirms your hypothesis that this woman is 'difficult'. The notion of the self-fulfilling prophecy is often linked in with attribution theory.

Attribution theory

You walk into a room and interrupt two of your colleagues who are involved in a heated argument. Emma is shouting aggressively at Sarah who appears to be upset and on the point of tears. You quickly walk out of the room, feeling rather embarrassed, but what do you think about what you have seen? It seems unlikely that you do not give it a second thought. You probably try to make sense of it in some way. Perhaps you know that these colleagues have a long-standing disagreement, or maybe you know that Jane has a very quick temper, perhaps you put the argument down to the stresses and strains that your colleagues are under. How you explain the situation will depend on the circumstances and what you already know about the people involved in the argument. What is most unlikely is that you will walk away from the situation and think no more about it. Almost certainly, you will try to make sense of what you have seen, in psychological jargon you will **attribute causes** in an attempt to explain the incident.

Psychologists have known about attribution for a long time. Heider (1944) believed that people were like naive scientists, analysing and actively trying to make sense of any situation they found themselves in and he was the first psychologist to describe the phenomena of **attribution of causality**. In very simple experiments using an animated film of balls moving towards each other, touching and then moving away again, he noted that people tended to describe this in a way that inferred that one ball was causing the other to move. This was interesting as there was nothing in the film to suggest that one action was causing another. The balls were only cartoon images and balls being inanimate objects cannot in themselves cause something to happen to another inanimate object. Heider reasoned that if we have a tendency to attribute causality to inanimate objects such as cartoon balls rolling about on a screen, we must also do this to animate objects such as people.

In further experiments Heider found this to be true, he also noted that we attribute causality in different ways. Sometimes we fix the explanation for the event on some quality within the individual and sometimes we explain the event in terms of something existing within the situation. He called this internal and external attribution respectively. It might be helpful to understand the distinction between internal and external attributions by going back to the example that began this section.

If having observed our two colleagues quarrelling we explained what we had seen by the quick temper of one of the participants, then we would have made an **internal** or **dispositional attribution**. That is, we would have attached the cause of the disagreement firmly on a quality existing in the character of one of the warring parties. If, on the other hand, we explained the argument in terms of the stresses that the two people were under we would have made an **external** or **situational attribution** and attributed the cause of the argument to an aspect of the situation. We will see later on that of the two kinds of attribution, we are more likely to make internal rather than external attributions, that is, we are more likely to blame the individual than the situation when it comes to explaining events.

Other researchers have built on Heider's ideas and expanded

attribution theory in an attempt to explain more precisely how we make attributions. The attributional or Lewinian Equation (named after Kurt Lewin a famous social psychologist, see Gilbert, 1995 for a fuller description) takes into account that any individual's behaviour (B) is partly influenced by the situation (S) and a person's disposition to act in a particular way (D). So that:

$$B = S + D$$

The process is more complicated than the example above indicates: there are many variables within any given situation that an onlooker may or may not take into consideration when making an attribution. How does he or she decide what to regard and what to ignore?

There are three theories that have attempted to analyse the attribution process in greater detail; correspondent inference theory (Jones and Davis, 1965), covariation theory (Kelley, 1967), and the causal schemata model (Kelley, 1972). Each of these attempts to analyse what exactly people are doing when they make attributions and they aim to predict how and what kind of attributions will be made. Although the three theories emphasise different aspects of attribution, they all make the assumption that attributions are made in logically consistent and reasoned ways. Only a brief account of the three models is given here, a more detailed account can be found in Hewstone and Fincham (1996).

The correspondent inference model (Jones and Davis, 1965) suggests that:

> *The goal of the attribution process is to infer that observed behaviour and the intention that produced it correspond to some underlying stable quality in the person or actor.*

(Hewstone and Fincham, 1996, p. 169)

In other words, when making attributions about what caused a situation, we try to put it down to some aspect of a person's character, hostility, for example. To do this we must first establish whether or not the actor intended to produce the effect they did. According to Jones and Davis we use information that helps us decide if the act was socially acceptable or not. If the act is deemed socially desirable then we gain little information about the actor. If, however, the act had socially undesirable consequences then we can make more inferences about the actor's personality and their intentions. To illustrate this let us return to the scenario described at the beginning of this section. If we believe that the observed aggressive behaviour on Jane's part is likely to lead to socially undesirable outcomes, such as being cold-shouldered by other colleagues then we will make the correspondent inference that the argument was due to the hostile and aggressive personality characteristics of Jane.

Kelley's covariation theory (1967) is used to predict attributions that are made when we are able to observe someone on numerous occasions and compare how they have behaved in the past and how other people behave towards them. According to this model, the person making an attribution does so on the basis of three pieces of information:

Consistency:	How the actor has behaved in the past.
Distinctiveness:	How the person behaves with others.
Consensus:	How others behave in the same situation.

Each of these three pieces of information about a situation can be either high or low. Consistency will be high if the actor has always behaved the same way in the past and low if the actor only behaves this way in a particular situation. Distinctiveness will be high if the actor only behaves this way with one person and low if she behaves this way with everyone. Consensus will be high if others behave in the same way in a given situation and low if it is only our actor who behaves in this way. We will make an internal or external attribution depending on how these three measures covary with each other and whether they measure high or low. This all gets rather confusing and by now you are probably completely mystified about how this model works. Let us go back to the argument between Emma and Sarah and see if we can cast some light on it.

We begin with the observation that Emma is verbally aggressive towards Sarah. According to Kelley's theory we consider:

Consistency:	Has Emma been aggressive towards Sarah in the past?
Distinctiveness:	Does Emma become aggressive towards other people or is it only Sarah?
Consensus:	Do other people behave aggressively towards Sarah?

We are likely to make an internal attribution and judge that the argument has been caused by Emma's aggressiveness if:

- consistency is high, that is, Emma has been aggressive towards Sarah in the past

- distinctiveness is high, that is, Emma gets aggressive with other people
- consensus is low, other people do not become aggressive with Sarah.

We are likely to make a situational or external attribution if:

- consistency is low, that is, Emma has not been aggressive towards Sarah in the past
- distinctiveness is low, that is, Emma does not become aggressive with others
- consensus is low, other people are not aggressive with Sarah.

Although Kelley suggested that people will use all three pieces of information equally, McArthur (1972) found that people were more likely to make internal rather than external attributions and use consistency more than either distinctiveness or consensus.

But what if we do not have the luxury of observing people on more than one occasion? We commonly make attributions based on a single observation. If we see someone who has collapsed in the street we might have to make a judgement about whether to offer help and must quickly decide if the person is ill, drunk or is merely play acting. To cope with the one-off situation Kelley proposed the causal schemata model (1972); he suggested that in such situations individuals have to rely on their knowledge (schemata) of how people behave in general. Making attributions based on single acts throws you back on your past experience of similar situations, stereotypes and implicit personality theory.

Even in a one-off situation there is often too much information for you to take in at once. For this reason, Kelley suggested that information is discounted if a plausible explanation for what you have observed is available (discounting principle). For example, if we see that the person who has collapsed is shabbily dressed with matted hair we might discount that they have had a heart attack and assume that they are simply another drunken down-and-out. The augmentation principle is applied if someone achieves something positive in the face of negative situational factors, for example, the achievement of a good grade in course work despite suffering from personal difficulties at home will be attributed to ability and other aspects of the situation will be ignored.

The three theories that have just been considered are all called normative models in that they attempt to explain how people should make attributions. All assume the process involves logical assessment of the available information leading to a rational decision. Although there is some evidence to support each of these theories (McArthur, 1972) research indicates that we often make attributions quickly and with very little information. In practice, attributions are often biased in ways that occur commonly and are both regular and predictable. Three different attributional biases have been described.

The fundamental attribution error

Although the phrase fundamental attribution error is still used for historical reasons, the word error is really a misnomer as it implies that there is a correct way of making attributions. This is something of a circular argument because the fundamental attribution error describes what people actually do in practice. The fundamental attribution error is only an error in as much as it is not what the normative models would predict, but it is what real people do in real (and laboratory) situations. The word bias is a much better descriptor of what this is all about.

In short, the fundamental attribution error states that when making attributions we are more likely to make internal (or dispositional) attributions than external (or situational) ones. We are more likely to attribute causality to an aspect of a person's personality than something within the situation. There is plenty of experimental evidence to support this, but we only have to look at the daily newspapers to see real life examples of it. If there is some sexual scandal surrounding an MP then the politician involved is labelled as faithless, unreliable, untrustworthy etc. Very rarely are the circumstances surrounding his or her misdemeanour considered. We are quick to label people and attribute responsibility to them personally with little or no consideration of any extenuating circumstances that may exist.

In midwifery practice it is important to be aware of this attributional bias. It is perhaps easier to put a 'difficult' client's behaviour down to an awkward personality rather than consider the situation and how this might be influencing what she does.

Actor/observer differences

It has been noted that people make different attributions depending on whether they are participants in a situation or merely observers. When we are participants we tend to make more situational attributions than if we are observers when the tendency is to make more dispositional attributions. It is difficult to know why this should be the case. Some researchers have suggested that it is to do with the amount of information that is available; when you are participating in a situation yourself you have more knowledge about both the situation and the participants, including yourself. You are more able to make an accurate attribution than if you are simply an observer when you tend to fall back on the fundamental attribution error.

Self-serving bias

This attributional bias works effectively to protect the ego, it describes the proclivity to make internal attributions when something positive happens to us and make external attributions when something goes wrong. For example, when we achieve a good mark in an assignment we give ourselves the credit for it, congratulating ourselves on our hard work and ability. When we only get a poor mark, we put our failure down to some aspect of the situation such as unfair questions, unrealistic deadlines, heavy workloads, biased marking and so on.

More recently, the self-serving bias has been found to exist at a group level and this has been called the group serving bias (Hewstone and Fincham, 1996). Evidence shows that we demonstrate attributional biases that protect group membership and emphasise differences between in-groups and out-groups. In-group successes are explained by invoking internal attributions and failures are blamed on external factors. For example, a group of disappointed football supporters might argue that their team only lost because the referee was unfair and turned a blind eye to the opposing team's errors. Had the team won, the explanation would have been that their team contained the most skilful footballers.

In the hospital setting I think we see this group serving tendency when professional groups close ranks to safeguard their member-ship, or when they compete with each in terms of expertise. Such attributional biases may act to protect group members and enhance the esteem of the group but they do little to protect the needs of clients who may well be caught in the middle of the warring factions.

Implications for midwifery practice

This chapter has discussed the human tendency to 'make sense' of social situations by making assumptions about people's personality characteristics and attributing causality. It has been argued that in most everyday situations people are good enough at this and cope well with the majority of social events they encounter. When meeting people for the first time or dealing with everyday situations things go reasonably smoothly, and this is probably true in the healthcare setting too.

However, here we might argue that there is a difference. The relationship between a health professional and a patient is not an equal one, there is an imbalance of power. The health professional has more expert knowledge than the client and will be in a position to make decisions about the client's management. Incorrect attributions can have far-reaching consequences for the client, something that might be less important in any other setting. Perhaps it helps to make more sense of this by illustrating it with a concrete example. Imagine that you are confronted with a pregnant woman who has been unable to give up smoking during her pregnancy. We know from the fundamental attribution error that we are more likely to put this down to a dispositional rather than a situational cause. You might be tempted to explain the woman's inability to control her addiction in terms of personal weakness, lack of self-control or not caring enough about the consequences of her behaviour on the unborn baby. But none of this might be true, there could be many situational factors in this client's life that have made it extremely difficult for her to break the habit. It is unlikely that the midwife has the time to find out about these and even if the woman herself tries to explain we might be tempted to put these down as 'excuses'. Similar dispositional attributions could be made to pregnant women who were very over-weight or who drank or took drugs during pregnancy.

Conclusion

The attributions that we make are almost bound to affect the way we treat women during pregnancy, labour and the postpartum period. Perhaps we will be less tolerant of them, more dismissive of their pain and discomfort and generally less empathetic to their situation. This will in turn influence the woman's behaviour, Gilbert puts this succinctly:

> *(What I think) affects (how I behave) which affects (what you think) which affects (how you behave) which affects (what I think).*

> (Gilbert, 1995, p. 126)

What can be done to avoid this kind of subtle influence on our behaviour? At first glance, this may seem like an impossible task, after all, midwives are only human and behave just like everyone else in this respect. It seems that there are two things that midwives and other health professionals can work on that can help them to avoid some of the worst pitfalls. Firstly, an awareness of the inter-personal perceptions and attribution processes that are at work in social situations is important. Although awareness in itself may not stop you making faulty attributions it is bound to help you to be more cognisant of what is happening in social situations. It may be possible for you to take steps to avoid the various attribution errors that have been discussed in this chapter. Secondly, you can practice consciously treating all clients as individuals. In my experience, the best way of doing this is to listen carefully to what clients are telling you (*Chapter 5*) and take the time to try to understand them. While I appreciate that this is not always easy when you are busy and have many people to deal with, it is important to avoid shorthand methods of summing people up which can lead to negative consequences for the client.

Finally, be wary of the group serving bias, while pride in-group membership is important do not let it stand in the way of your professional judgement.

References

Asch S (1946) Forming impressions of personality. *J Abnorm Soc Psychol* **41**: 258–90

Fiske ST (1993) Social cognition and social perception. *Annu Rev Psychol* **44**: 155–94

Gilbert DT (1995) Attribution and interpersonal perception. In: Tesser A, ed. *Advanced Social Psychology*. McGraw Hill, New York: 99–146

Heider F (1944) Social perception and phenomenal causality. *Psychol Rev* **52**: 358–78

Heider F (1958) *The Psychology of Interpersonal Relations*. Wiley, New York

Hewstone M, Fincham F (1996) Attribution theory and research: Basic issues and application. In: Hewstone M, Stroebe W, Stephenson G, eds. *Introduction to Social Psychology*. 2nd edn. Blackwell, Oxford: 168–204

Jones EE, Davis KE (1965) From acts to dispositions: the attribution process in person perception. In: Berkowitz L, ed. *Advances in Experimental Social Psychology* (Vol 2). Academic Press, New York

Kelley HH (1967) Attribution theory in social psychology. In: Levine D, ed. *Nebraska symposium on motivation*. University of Nebraska Press, Lincoln: vol 15, 192–238

Kelley HH (1972) Causal schemata and the attribution process. In: Jones EE, Kanouse DE, Kelley HH, Nisbeth RE, Valius S, Weiner B, eds. *Attribution: Perceiving the causes of behaviour*. General Learning Press, Morristown, NJ: 151–74

Pennington DC (1982) Witnesses and their testimony: Effects of ordering on juror's verdicts. *J Appl Soc Psychol* **12**(4): 318–33

Pennington DC (1986) *Essential Social Psychology*. Edward Arnold, London

Pennington DC, Gillen K, Hill P (1999) *Social Psychology*. Arnold, London

Rosenthal R, Jacobsen LF (1968) *Pygmalion in the Classroom*. Holt, Rinehard and Winston, New York

Zebrowitz LA (1990) *Social Perception*. Pacific Grove, Brooks/Cole, CA

5

Communication: what you say is not always what you mean

Human ingenuity seems to be developing increasingly sophisticated ways of enabling us to communicate with each other more quickly and efficiently. Modern technology now makes it possible to make contact with someone on the other side of the globe almost as easily as we can communicate with a colleague in the next office. Fast and efficient communication is demanded in the form of news and current events so that now more than ever before we have up to the minute accurate information about what is happening in far-flung corners of the world. Unfortunately the existence of sophisticated technology does not solve the problems of human interaction in face-to-face situations, which still seem to be fraught with the risk of misunderstanding and misinterpretation. Although as humans we spend a large part of every day interacting with others, there is a great deal of individual variation in our ability to communicate effectively.

While good communication skills are important for everyone, they are particularly salient for health professionals. The way information is given to people who may be in pain, anxious and vulnerable, can have a major impact on how healthcare information is received and whether it is acted on (Kreps *et al*, 1995). As a midwife you will undoubtedly encounter many situations that will involve the communication of difficult information to women and their families. Maybe you will have to tell a labouring mother who really wants a vaginal delivery that she has to have a Caesarean section, or perhaps you will have to explain that the labour is not progressing as it should. On occasions you may have to give worse news, perhaps there has been a stillbirth or some serious medical complication during labour. How do you tackle these situations? What communication skills do you employ to ensure that you get the message across in a way that is sensitive to the feelings and needs of the recipient and yet still enables you to do your job?

This chapter considers why communication skills are particularly important for health professionals and what psychological theory can contribute to the professional development of the midwife in this aspect of health care. I do not give practical exercises in communication skills. The intention is to give you an understanding of the elements that make for a good communicator so that you can begin to be more self-aware about your own communicative abilities and put this into practice in your professional (and personal) life. If you would like a book that gives more practical skills training there are many good ones available on the market (Williams, 1997).

The importance of good communication skills for health professionals

What makes a good communicator? Think of someone that you know who has good communication skills. What is it about their style that is effective? In general, a good communicator is able to:

- deliver a clear message and get their point across
- take into account the receiver of the message and tailor it appropriately so that they do not talk down to people
- use appropriate non-verbal gestures/tone of voice etc
- respond sensitively and reflectively to others verbal and non-verbal cues.

Thompson (1994) points out that communication in healthcare settings is unique because of the 'life and death' nature of much of the interaction. This means that good communication skills are essential for anyone involved in working in these situations. As Dickson *et al* (1997) comment, 'effective communication lies at the heart of successful healthcare delivery'.

Although communication skills can be seen as being of crucial importance in healthcare settings, health professionals often receive little or no training in this area. It has been recognised for many years that there have been deficiencies in communication between health professionals and patients and yet things do not seem to have changed a great deal. According to Numann (1988, quoted in Dickson *et al*, 1997, p. 10):

> *We have failed to teach our students the interpersonal skills which will enable them to effectively communicate with the patient, to consider the patient's needs and wishes, to encourage the patient to appropriately participate in their care, and to treat the patient with respect and dignity.*

It is frequently assumed that good communication skills are a natural gift, you either have or lack the ability. Often, little by way of training is given to health professionals, resulting in many short-comings in communication between patients and health professionals. In fact, the majority of research indicates that most patient dissatisfaction has some aspect of poor communication at its root and nursing, midwifery and health visiting have all been found wanting in this regard.

In a review of a number of studies, Davis and Fallowfield (1993) conclude that communication skills of health professionals are deficient in many areas, including:

1. Failure to greet the patient appropriately, to introduce themselves, and to explain their actions.
2. Failure to elicit easily available information, especially major worries and expectations.
3. Acceptance of imprecise information and the failure to seek clarification.
4. Failure to check the health professional's understanding of the situation against the patient's.
5. Failure to encourage questions or to answer them appropriately.
6. Neglect of covert and overt cues provided verbally or otherwise by the patient.
7. Avoidance of information about the personal, family and social situation, including problems in these areas.
8. Failure to elicit information about the patient's feelings and perceptions of the illness.
9. Directive style with closed questions predominating, frequent interruptions and failure to let the patient talk spontaneously.
10. Focusing too quickly without hypothesis testing.
11. Failure to provide information adequately about diagnosis, treatment, side-effects, or prognosis, or to check subsequent understanding.
12. Failure to understand from the patient's viewpoint and hence to be supportive.
13. Poor reassurance.

Such poor communication skills lead not only to patient dissatisfaction, but also to non-compliance with advice and treatment, inaccurate diagnosis because the appropriate information has not been elicited and poor physical and psychological outcome.

In essence, many health professionals tend not to listen to their clients, they assume a position of power which protects them but inhibits the patient from asking questions. Clinicians frequently construe themselves as experts in relation to diagnosis and treatment, this then overgeneralises to all aspects of the patient and their relationship. The implicit assumption is that the expert knows what he or she is doing and that the patient has little to offer the debate.

In terms of midwifery practice, it is important to remember that much of what the midwife does in her professional role contravenes normal rules of interaction. When doing a vaginal examination, delivering a baby or helping a woman to breastfeed her new baby, you are dealing intimately with areas of her body that are not generally exposed to strangers. In addition, the power balance in the interaction is very one-sided. While you are fully dressed, she may well be only partially clothed or in her nightwear, so the way in which you use both verbal and non-verbal aspects of communication in these situations is critically important and can do much to alleviate embarrassment and put the woman at ease. This will have positive benefits both in terms of enabling the client to ask pertinent questions and in providing an environment where the midwife can give important information regarding health care to the mother. It may also positively influence a woman's experience of labour.

No health professional can be complacent about communication. Good communication is essential for patient satisfaction and there is always room for greater understanding of the elements that comprise good communication skills and the practice of these skills in healthcare settings.

What do we mean by communication anyway?

'Communication' is one of those words like 'stress' that is used frequently in modern society and yet is difficult to define precisely. We can, however, describe what communication involves. At its most basic level communication must include:

- something that is to be communicated or a message
- a person (or machine) that gives the message
- a person (or machine) who receives the message.

When we consider human communication we must also take into account the content of the message and the effect that it has upon the listener.

In addition, interpersonal communication is usually purposeful. In other words, people communicate with each other in order to get things done in the world. It is also transactional, when two or more people engage in communicative acts they act as both senders and receivers of messages.

Face-to-face communication involves verbal and non-verbal signals. Verbal communication is to a large degree under conscious control, because we are able to choose what words to say during an interaction. The verbal component of communication is always accompanied by certain non-verbal elements of speech such as pitch and intonation. Without these, spoken language would simply be a boring monotone and these elements add musicality and rhythm to the spoken word. Non-verbal components of speech also give the listener information about the emotional content of the message. These non-verbal components of language are not as easily controlled as the verbal element and may give us away if they do not correspond with the words that are being spoken. For example, saying 'I hate you' with a soft tone of voice while gazing into someone's eyes probably means the exact opposite. The speed and loudness of speech also has communicative value for the listener as does the register we use, that is, the degree of formality or informality.

Other non-verbal elements of communication bring into play different aspects of the body. This is sometimes referred to as 'body language' and includes:

- facial expression
- gaze and pupil dilation
- gestures and other bodily movements
- posture
- bodily contact
- spatial behaviour
- clothes and other aspects of appearance
- smell.

(taken from Argyle, 1988)

Researchers have found that non-verbal communication (NVC) not only complements and supports language but also plays a highly significant role in human interaction (Argyle, 1988). Like the non-verbal vocalisations we have just described, these aspects of communication are much more difficult to control at a conscious level. Some can be brought under conscious control, for example, we can choose whether to make eye contact with someone or how close we stand to them, but many are automatic responses over which we either have no control or we find difficult to control. We cannot prevent pupil dilation when we look at someone we find sexually attractive, but we may manage partially to suppress a grimace of disgust if we are confronted with something that we find distasteful.

In everyday situations we use both verbal and non-verbal communication in face-to-face interaction. These two aspects of interpersonal interaction generally dovetail smoothly with the non-verbal aspects of communication acting to emphasise and complement our words. There are times when the two do not always correspond, as when we say something that we do not really mean and our body language gives us away. Let us look more closely at both non-verbal and verbal communication.

Non-verbal communication

We saw earlier that communication is made up of both verbal and non-verbal components. Non-verbal communication (NVC) includes hand gestures, body posture and facial expressions. Quite often we are not aware of transmitting information to others via non-verbal cues, but it is possible to use what we know of NVC deliberately and it is often taught as part of communication skills, for example, adopting an 'open' posture rather than a 'closed' one. This section of the chapter discusses what psychologists understand about non-verbal aspects of interaction and the influence that this has upon communication.

We use NVC:

- as an aid to speech
- instead of speech
- to signal attitudes
- to signal emotional states.

NVC plays a significant role in nearly all social interactions. Although it would be extremely difficult to communicate complex messages via non-verbal means alone, the emotional content of any communication is usually transmitted primarily via the non-verbal channel. Health professionals need to be aware of the non-verbal aspects of patient communication as this is a useful indicator of the emotional state of the individual. Sensitivity to non-verbal cues may help to prevent many misunderstandings and feelings of patient dissatisfaction.

The face

Facial expression

Although we use the whole of the body in non-verbal communication perhaps the face is the part of the body that is most important. We tend to look at other people's faces while they are speaking and their expression and the amount of eye contact they make with us influences the way that the message is received by the listener. Facial expressions give us strong clues about the emotions and feelings that the other person is experiencing. There are six facial expressions that seem to be universally recognised across cultures. These are; disgust, anxiety, sadness, happiness, surprise and anger (Ekman, 1992) and even small infants appear to be able to demonstrate these emotions in their facial expressions (Rozin *et al*, 1994).

This does not mean that these are the only emotions that can be demonstrated in the face. It is possible to have infinite combinations such as anxiety tinged with sadness and anger linked with disgust and surprise. In general, we are not as easily able to identify these combinations and cross-cultural differences may be more apparent.

In fact, humans are very skilled at recognising and interpreting facial expressions and we need very few cues to do it. The following is an exercise I often use with groups of students to convince them of this. *Figure 5.1* shows a series of schematic faces. As you can see, these 'faces' are made up of only a few lines, dots and curves, hardly faces at all, and yet I am sure you will easily be able to recognise the emotions expressed on each.

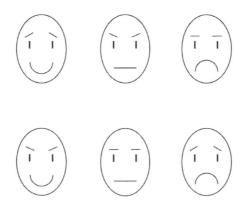

Figure 5.1: Schematic faces — can you recognise the emotions?

In face-to-face situations recognising emotions may be more difficult, this is because we often express combinations of emotions rather than the six simple ones that Ekman describes and we may well try to disguise our facial expressions. Often the rules of social interaction demand that certain emotions are not expressed. For example, it is rude to look disgusted at a dinner party even if you are presented with a type of food that you cannot stomach (eg. snails, sheep's eyes) and you may try to cover up your involuntary revulsion in some way. Boredom is another emotion that is shown clearly in the face but one that we often work hard to suppress.

In the midwifery setting it is important to be aware that both you and the mother-to-be might be attempting to control your facial expressions so as not to give away certain emotions. The mother may be trying hard not to show that she is afraid, you as the midwife may at times be attempting to hide your feelings of panic or even disgust. Sometimes health professionals feel that they should not show sadness when some tragedy occurs, but I am not convinced that this is necessarily good practice and may well come across to the client that you just do not care. The midwife really needs to be sensitive to facial expressions particularly when they appear to contradict the verbal component of the communication. In these circumstances it is always worthwhile making sure that you have understood correctly, this may well give the mother the opportunity she needs to tell you what she is really feeling.

Eye contact

The amount of eye contact we make with another person varies along a number of dimensions and most cultures have quite complex rituals regarding this. In general, we tend to look at people that we like and avoid the gaze of those that we do not. We expect others to look at us while we are talking to them and will assume that they are bored or uninterested if they continually look away. During a conversation we look at the speaker to signal that we wish to take a turn and look away to signal that we have finished saying what we wanted to say.

If we look at someone for too long, this is regarded as rude or even hostile. Most of us feel uncomfortable if someone appears to be staring at us and might take steps to avoid the person's gaze (Ellsworth and Carlsmith, 1973). It is quite interesting to try the following exercise. Make eye contact with a friend or colleague and see how long you can hold each other's gaze without one of you looking away. This is quite a difficult thing to do, the chances are that you will be able to look longer at someone you know very well, but it is surprising how uncomfortable this exercise can make you feel. Making eye contact with people is an essential part of good communication. If you made no eye contact with a woman during her labour, she would undoubtedly feel that you were uncaring or indifferent. However, there is a fine line to be drawn and making too much eye contact can be inappropriate and even threatening, especially when you are in close proximity to someone.

Pupil dilation

It is obviously within our conscious control to increase or decrease the amount of eye contact that we make with someone in a face-to-face interaction, but pupil dilation is a physical response over which we have no control. This response occurs if we gaze at someone whom we find attractive. In general, we are not aware of this happening at a conscious level, although it seems that there is some recognition at a subconscious level. In a classic experiment men were shown two photographs of the same woman, in one of the photographs the pupils had been artificially enlarged and this photograph was consistently rated as being more attractive than the other. This indicates that we do respond to pupil dilation, but it is not something that we need to be concerned about as there is little we can do to alter or influence the situation.

Posture, gesture and physical proximity

Just as we need minimal cues to recognise the emotions expressed by facial expressions we are also skilled at understanding the meaning of a person's body posture. If an individual is sitting hunched over with downcast eyes and their head in their hands then we assume that they are feeling sad and depressed. On the other hand, someone standing with a very open posture would be likely to be expressing a more positive emotion; similarly, someone sitting up and looking alert during a conversation would be indicating that they are interested in what was being said, while someone slumped in the chair staring out of the window would be signalling boredom.

Figure 5.2 shows some matchstick men in various postures. Can you guess what each is 'feeling'? Get someone else to do the exercise and then compare your results, you will be surprised at the level of agreement.

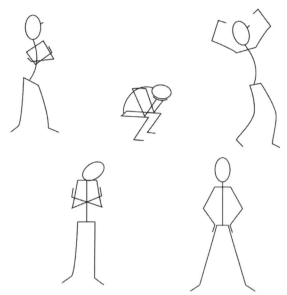

Figure 5.2: Matchstick men — what emotions do the body postures portray?

The hands

The hands are one part of the body that are particularly important in communication. We use hand gestures all the time to emphasise and add weight to the words that we utter. (If you are not convinced about this, try carrying out a conversation while sitting on your hands — it feels very strange.) There are quite marked cross-cultural differences in the use of gesture. For example, the Italians tend to use them more frequently and more expansively than the British, but there are also particular differences in the meaning of more stereotyped gestures which one needs to be aware of. I am not an expert on this, but I do know that the gesture we use to signal OK, the thumb and first finger touching to form a circle and the other fingers raised, is an extremely rude and offensive sign in some parts of the world.

Cultural differences

This raises an important point; as there are many different rules regarding NVC across the world it is important for any midwife or health professional to find out about these when working with different ethnic groups to avoid causing offence. Take proximity, for example. In Britain we tend not to stand close to people unless we know them very well, and may feel uncomfortable when forced to stand close to strangers in a crowded lift. In these circumstances we avoid making eye contact and this is why everyone stares so intently at the door or the sign just above the door showing which floor the lift is on. This is not true in other cultures, where the norm is for people to stand or sit closer. There is a funny story that illustrates this point, but is no doubt apocryphal, about a meeting between two business-men, one British and one Arabic. Following the proximity rules of his culture the Arab moved quite close to the British businessman. He however, found this uncomfortable and moved away. The Arab moved closer once more, while the British man moved a step or two away. In this manner the two of them were in constant motion around the room, both feeling that they could not really get on with the job in hand because they were not standing at the right distance to each other.

It is important to recognise that in your role as a midwife, you inevitably contravene the proximity rules of any culture. Part of your job involves standing extremely close to people and touching parts of their bodies that are not usually exposed to relative strangers. This means that you have to be particularly sensitive about the use of non-verbal communication and need to monitor both your own and the client's behaviour to ensure that everyone is comfortable with the situation and there is minimal embarrassment.

I hope to have highlighted two things in this brief discussion of NVC. Firstly, even if we occasionally feel that we are socially inept, we are all skilled at reading the non-verbal cues of others, it is our ability to do this that enables everyday social interactions to unfold smoothly. Secondly, health professionals need to be particularly sensitive to non-verbal cues and this applies to their own, as well as those of clients, if there is to be effective communication. Because the non-verbal content of the communication is less under conscious control it is often a more 'honest' response and provides a window into the patient's feelings. By being alert to this, misunderstandings may well be averted. In addition, the midwife must be careful about her own non-verbal cues. Failing to smile and make eye contact when meeting a pregnant woman for the first time may well get the relationship off on the wrong foot and lead to negative feelings on the part of both mother and midwife. It is obviously worthwhile to practice self-awareness in the use of NVC and maybe even (if you are feeling brave) ask colleagues to observe you interacting with clients and make constructive comments about your skills.

Verbal communication

In modern society we are bathed in language from the moment we wake until the time we go to sleep. We are bombarded with the spoken and written word through radio, television, newspapers, magazines and now the internet. If you are unconvinced of the truth of this, try the following brief exercise. Think about a normal working day in your life and then consider how much of the time is spent in communicating with others, talking, listening, giving information and exchanging ideas. If you spend a few minutes on this exercise you might be surprised by the proportion of time that you spend engaged in acts of communication. In fact, talk will probably be a part of every interaction that you have with other people.

Every human society has language; it is probably the major reason why as a species we have been so successful. We can use language to express complex ideas and concepts and pass these on to the next generation thus getting rid of the necessity of reinventing the wheel (or the computer) every few decades. All known languages are highly evolved systems which use symbols (words), which have meaning (semantics) in various combinations (grammar) to represent objects and events in the world. This allows us to communicate our perceptions about our environment to others and to share personal experience: but communication is not simply about the spoken word. As we have already seen, we also use the non-verbal component of language such as tone, speed, volume and emphasis to signal our emotional state and add emphasis to our words.

Language is made up of several components, phonology, semantics, syntax and pragmatics. Phonology refers to different sounds that make up any given language; semantics refers to the meaning that each word has, while syntax reflects the rules that we use to combine words in a meaningful way. Pragmatics refers to the social rules that govern the use of appropriate language. This also includes register which relates to the formality or informality of the language we choose to use in a given setting. Every human language in the world contains these components although the particular sounds that make up any language, word meaning and the rules used to combine words vary from one language to another.

All of these elements of language come together in every communicative act in which we engage, but we use language with so little effort that we are rarely aware of its complexity; and yet it is extremely difficult to reproduce. No other species is able to communicate in such a way, and people are still trying to programme computers to talk like humans (Aitchison, 1998).

Language is fundamentally a social activity. It is interesting to reflect whether we would have any use for language if we suddenly found ourselves stranded alone on a desert island. Would we talk to ourselves? As the main purpose of language is to communicate with others I suspect that eventually we would cease to use language until we found another person or animal to whom we could talk. As adults we have a sophisticated understanding of the appropriate use of language in social situations and change our verbal utterances accordingly. What is appropriate language at a party, for example, will not be acceptable at a job interview or in a meeting at work. In a relaxed social setting we use sloppier language, slang terms and perhaps refer to incidences in a rather vague way, knowing that others share our knowledge of these events. Regional accents may become broader and in some cases regional dialects may be used. In formal settings we use more formal language and are careful about the grammaticality of what we say. Explanations are more specific and we might modify and tone down regional accents and dialects.

There have been various theories put forward that attempt to explain what is being achieved when talk is going on within a social context; the assumption being that talk always serves some kind of purpose. Even talk that on the surface appears unimportant may be helping us to forge and maintain social relationships with others. Hymes (1967, quoted in Halliday, 1978) is one of those who has attempted to explain every relevant feature of any social interaction that includes verbal language. I will spend some time discussing Hymes' model as I believe it really helps to give a fuller understanding of the complexity of talk and its intensely social nature. As you read, you may notice that the first letter of each heading rather ingeniously spells the word 'speaking'.

Setting and scene

The setting embraces the time, place and physical circumstance in which the speech occurs; the scene designates how an occasion is culturally defined and perceived. Speech acts may define the scene as when someone says, 'Let's play cards' and may be judged appropriate or inappropriate to a scene. For example, in an antenatal clinic a woman would not be surprised by a male doctor asking her to lie down so that he can feel her tummy. However, in a supermarket the same request by a male would be regarded as very inappropriate behaviour. The setting and scene are to a large extent culturally defined and we learn through childhood what language is appropriate for each social scenario.

Participants

These are all the people who make up any given setting and scene and who are involved in the communication in some way. They may be active participants engaged in giving and receiving messages, but participants can also include onlookers who are passive participants of the interaction.

Ends

Hymes assumes that every speech act has an intended outcome, ie. something that the participant is trying to achieve through the interaction. As a midwife your intended outcome in talking to a woman in labour may be to calm her down so that you can discuss her birth plan with her. If you manage to do this then you will have achieved your goal, however the outcome of the interaction could be something that you did not intend at all (she might become even more distressed and refuse to discuss her birth plan with you). Successful communicators will achieve their goals more often than not.

Act sequence

The form and content of the message are tightly interdependent. The way in which something is said, angrily, cheerfully and so on becomes an integral part of what is said and cannot be separated from it.

Key

This refers to the tone or manner of a speech act which might be mocking, polite or solemn etc. This may depend to some extent on the mood of the speaker but will also derive from the social situation. At a funeral, for example, the key will be solemn, a mocking or jolly tone would be felt to be inappropriate. A serious tone would also be adopted when giving someone bad news.

Instrumentalities

We can use different instruments to communicate with each other. Most often we use oral communication but we can also use the written word and various technical apparatus such as the telephone or e-mail. Instrumentalities also includes the languages and dialects with which we choose to communicate.

Norms of interaction and interpretation

All rules governing speaking are normative and change from time to time; speech acts may have features that have community meaning. For example, a falling tone and lengthened vowel for saying 'yes' may signal disagreement and uncertainty, rather than agreement. It is important to be aware that such norms of interaction and inter-pretation vary from culture to culture and even within groups of people who share the same language can lead to misunderstandings.

Genres

These are clearly marked categories such as verbal games, poems and story-telling. Other genre could include such things as formal lectures where the tone tends to be formal and the language more technical. In general, we have an understanding of what is expected in certain kinds of genre, we would be surprised if during a lecture the lecturer began using slang and taboo words and a language style that was more appropriate for chatting to friends in the pub.

This list demonstrates, more than anything else, the fact that language does not simply consist of the words that are spoken. Many different elements contribute towards the meaning of an utterance and not just the utterance itself. The way language is interpreted by others will depend on many of these components. For example, consider the sentence, 'I think you are seriously ill'. If such a phrase were uttered by a doctor during a medical consultation then the addressee would be forgiven for thinking that they were about to hear some bad news. If the same sentence is said in a joking tone of voice at a party the utterance takes on a completely different complexion. The interpretation depends on the social setting, the non-verbal cues such as tone of voice, body language and who is speaking to whom.

The problem with jargon

Generally, those engaged in communicative acts in medical settings have a reasonably clear idea of the roles that they are playing and what kind of language is acceptable in such contexts. It is not easy to keep lines of communication open if health professionals do not take their audience into account and continue to talk in medical jargon, completely failing to recognise that the people to whom they are talking may not fully understand what is being said. This does not mean that they are either stupid or ignorant, but simply that they do not have access to this kind of language. As a violinist I might talk of playing a piece of music allargando or using martele or spicatto bowing. If you do not play a stringed instrument such terms may mystify you. This does not mean that you lack intelligence, simply that you are not familiar with the words. I could very quickly explain what they mean and then you would have little difficulty understanding. Jargon is insidious because the terms quickly become familiar to those who frequently use them, making it easy to overlook the fact that others do not share the same knowledge.

> *In particular, practitioners who possess a deeper knowledge of medical issues than their patients, must relate necessary details to the patients in a manner understandable to those patients. For example, the very use of specific medical terminology (which may well be second nature to the practitioners) during a given encounter contributes little to patient understanding when patients do not even know the correct meaning of the terminology.*

(Beck and Ragan, 1995, p. 77)

In medical settings, when people may be apprehensive anyway it is essential to check that what is said is fully understood. Even when medical terminology is not used confusion can occur. I am reminded of a story a midwife once told me. While doing a scan on a pregnant woman she had commented in a rather vague way that she could not find the baby's head, meaning of course that the baby was lying in such a way that the head could not be observed on the scan. The poor woman left with the impression that the baby she was carrying had no head. It was not until the next day that she came back to the midwife asking for clarification. Although at one level the story is amusing, the anguish experienced by the mother does not bear thinking about. Misunderstandings of this kind can cause untold anxiety and can only be avoided by the practitioner constantly checking for clues from the client that they have understood fully the implications of what has been said and done during an encounter.

Sutherland *et al* (1991) carried out a study in which cancer patients were asked to put a numerical value to words like 'rare', 'likely', 'possible' and 'occasionally'. These are terms that are often used to describe risks to patients on the basis of which decisions about treatment may need to be made. Rather disturbingly, the study found that there was little consensus about the numerical value that these terms represented and participants attached different values to the terms when they were presented in different formats (paper and pencil tests as opposed to computer). The researchers rightly question whether under these circumstances, when these words are used, patients' consent can truly be regarded as being 'informed'.

Hadlow and Pitts (1991) suggested that health professionals and lay people may use the same terms but in different ways thereby creating misunderstandings. They took a range of medical and psychological terms such as 'schizophrenia', 'epilepsy' and 'coronary thrombosis' and asked medical practitioners, nurses, health support workers and patients to choose from a number of definitions. The findings showed that there were clear differences of understanding between the health professionals and patients. Such differences could well lead to poor communication which might in turn cause patient dissatisfaction and a failure to comply with advice.

In the past, jargon and medicalised terminology may have been used in front of patients as a deliberate strategy to distance professionals emotionally and make them appear more knowledgeable. However, this does not contribute in any positive way to good relationships between the health professional and client or to patient satisfaction. In any communicative act in whatever setting, it is essential to take the addressee into consideration and modify language accordingly. For the vast majority of time we do this quite naturally, without really thinking about it. For example, you would not talk to a five-year-old child in the same way as you would talk to another adult. Likewise, it is important for midwives and other health professionals to check with pregnant and labouring women that they fully understand what is being said to them and avoid as much as possible the use of obscure jargon terms. It goes without saying that this should not be done in a patronising way while keeping the communication as clear as possible.

In addition, care should be taken to monitor the non-verbal aspects of speech, such as speed, pitch and loudness. If you talk too quickly then the client may not be able to take in what you are saying, on the other hand, speaking too slowly may appear condescending. Similarly, if you talk too softly the client may not be able to hear you and your tone might indicate that you are lacking in confidence about what you are saying. Speaking too loudly might appear aggressive and intimidating. How do you get it right, how do you strike the right balance? There are several practical things that you could do to help develop your skills in this area:

❖ Observe colleagues who you feel strike the right balance when talking to clients and try to model your behaviour on theirs.

❖ Ask colleagues to give you objective feedback and try to adapt your behaviour accordingly.

❖ Try to be sensitive to the clients that you talk to, do not just keep talking at them but look for signs of confusion and give them a chance to ask questions.

❖ Pause regularly so that the client can take their turn in the conversation and make a comment; this can help you to check whether or not they are following what you are saying.

Beck and Ragan (1995) studied interaction between nurses and women during a gynaecological examination. In this study they found that certain strategies on the part of the practitioner helped the interaction, in particular, the use of humour and some degree of self-disclosure enabled women to ask questions and participate more fully in the examination. The next section on basic counselling skills also gives some useful suggestions about communicating with others.

Basic counselling skills

Skills that have been developed for use in counselling situations can be enormously helpful in healthcare settings, and can be used in combination with language and NVC to enhance effective communication between the health professional and the client. Using simple counselling skills does not make you a counsellor but it does enable you to demonstrate to clients that you are actively listening to their concerns and attempting to understand what they are trying to say. This is conducive to good communication and patient satisfaction. The skills use a mixture of both verbal and non-verbal behaviours, including:

- attending
- active listening
- positive regard
- non-judgemental attitudes.

To find out more about these basic counselling skills both Egan (2001) and Nelson-Jones (2000) provide very good introductions to basic counselling that are only briefly sketched here.

Attending

We generally know when someone is not really interested in a conversation. They may look bored, or even yawn. Their eyes look glazed, their body is slightly turned away from us and they may make little or no eye contact. Perhaps they respond verbally in a rather half-hearted way with a flat tone of voice. We know that this sort of behaviour is not very encouraging and if we are sensitive we either end the interaction or try to do something to engage the person we are talking to more fully. When working with clients it is important to use verbal and non-verbal cues to indicate that we are, in fact, attending to what they are saying. This might involve the use of continuation messages such as nodding or saying 'mmm' and 'right' or 'I understand', looking alert, leaning towards them and making eye contact. It also includes mirroring their facial expressions to some extent. When you attend to someone in this way it has a wonderful effect on them. They begin to relax and are more likely to tell you what is really concerning them, and they feel positive because you are showing all the signs of being genuinely interested in what they have to say.

You can practice attending in situations outside the healthcare setting. Try it at home with your family and friends. Although it may feel awkward to you at first, I can almost guarantee that the person you practice on will not notice, but will simply feel very positive about the outcome of the conversation.

Active listening

In general, we are very bad at listening to what others are telling us. In normal everyday conversations we are rarely totally alert to what is being said to us. Perhaps it is because we are engaged in other activities when people are talking to us, more often than not we are busy composing a reply in our heads and thinking about our contribution to the conversation, sometimes before the person who is speaking has even finished their turn. In your work as a midwife perhaps your mind is actively thinking about medical matters while you are talking to a pregnant woman or maybe you are anxious about your next appointment and what you have to do there.

Listening actively to another person is not easy. It means that you have to give your full attention so that you can concentrate completely on what is being said to you. It also means that you must suspend the chatter within your own head and resist the temptation to jump in with your own contribution. I think active listening is particularly difficult for people who are used to giving others advice, but it is essential if you are going to understand fully what the client is telling you. Again, you can try out active listening with family and friends. Listen without interrupting and then demonstrate your understanding of what has been said by reflecting back or maybe asking for clarification, for example, 'So, am I right in thinking that you would prefer a homebirth but are worried that something might go wrong?'

Active listening does not mean that you should let someone go on and on without interruption. You will need to stop people to make sure that you have understood them, but active listening does mean that you do your best to understand from the client's perspective what it is that they are trying to convey.

Positive regard

This is a term that has been taken from Carl Rogers' 'Client-centred therapy' (1980), and has been adopted into many approaches to counselling. The idea is that the therapist must take a positive attitude towards the person they are counselling and reflect this in their interaction with them. This is not always easy to do in practice. You will be aware that in normal social situations there are people you meet with whom you easily strike up a positive exchange. It may be because you find them attractive or interesting and it is relatively simple to respond in a friendly and easy manner. You do not have to pretend to like them because you do and this will be reflected in all aspects of your verbal and non-verbal communication. Alternatively, there are people to whom you take an immediate dislike and simply cannot feel anything positive about. Once again your feelings about them will reflect in your verbal and non-verbal interactions, you may avoid eye contact or adopt a hostile or defensive posture and smile infrequently.

Rogers argues that every human being deserves to be regarded in a positive way by others, regardless of their personal attributes. He believed that within all of us is the potential for psychological growth and lack of positive regard in childhood is the cause of many subsequent adult problems. Indeed, he makes the point that people who receive positive regard from others can grow and develop and achieve their full potential.

As a midwife you are not attempting to engage in therapy with women, but by trying to show positive regard for them you will undoubtedly make a difference to their experience of maternity care. When people experience positive regard, they feel valued and positive about themselves, this has the effect of increasing their self-confidence and may well help them to feel more in control of the situation (see the chapters on pregnancy and labour for a fuller discussion of control; *Chapters 6* and *7*). It is also likely to increase their trust in the person who is giving the positive regard, which will inevitably benefit both the woman and the midwife.

Non-judgemental attitude

In *Chapter 3* we discussed the issue of prejudice and how this can have a deleterious effect on the relationship between health professionals and their clients. Taking a non-judgemental attitude is part of giving the mother positive regard. It requires that you become aware of what your prejudices are and attempt to suspend them, at least during the time that you are interacting with the person you feel prejudiced against. It also means that you must try not to make judgements or assumptions about clients because of the way that they are dressed, or present themselves, by the way that they speak or behave.

Previous chapters noted how easy it is to come to incorrect judgements about people because of the way that they behave and we frequently disregard reasons for why they may be behaving in that manner. Midwives are only human and have just as many prejudices and preconceptions about groups of people as anyone else. Some common prejudices that student midwives have discussed in lectures were described in *Chapter 3*. I am sure that there are many more that I have missed, but as a midwife your prejudices can have a major impact on how a woman experiences her antenatal care or the birth of her baby. It is particularly important that you try to avoid your attitudes getting in the way of the interaction.

There is no doubt that taking a non-judgemental attitude and using positive regard will improve communication in the midwifery setting, which will have a positive impact on patient satisfaction and result in a better working environment for everyone.

Application to midwifery practice

I hope that this chapter has left you in no doubt about the importance of good communication in midwifery practice. There is now such a large body of research that indicates that patient dissatisfaction is largely caused by poor communication, that the health professional should take their own communicative abilities very seriously. By trying to be sensitive to what people are telling you and by being aware of your own verbal and non-verbal messages you can go a long way to improving patient satisfaction.

Conclusion

As a health professional working regularly with people who are anxious and/or in pain, good communication skills are absolutely essential.

You might be feeling overwhelmed by the complexity of communication. It is important to remember two things; firstly, you are already a skilled communicator and have been since the age of three or four. You have all the skills you need — you are simply trying to improve them so that you are better able to cope with the kind of sensitive situations that your work often demands. Secondly, this chapter is only a very brief introduction to different ideas about communication. Further study and lots of practice are required. It is certainly worthwhile spending time developing your skills in this area, as it will undoubtedly bear fruit in terms of patient satisfaction.

References

Aitchinson J (1998) *The Articulate Mammal*. 4th edn. Routledge, London
Argyle M (1988) *Bodily Communication*. 2nd edn. Routledge, London

Beck CS, Ragan SL (1995) The impact of relational activities on the accomplishment of practitioner and patient goals in the gynecological examination. In: Kreps GL, O'Hair D, eds. *Communication and Health Outcomes*. Hampton Press, Cresskill, New Jersey: 73–85

Davis H, Fallowfield L (1993) Counselling and communication in health care: The current situation. In: Davis H, Fallowfield L, eds. *Counselling and Communication in Health Care*. John Wiley, Chichester

Dickson D, Hargie O, Morrow N (1997) *Communication Skills Training for Health Professionals*. 2nd edn. Chapman and Hall, London

Egan G (2001) *The Skilled Helper*. 7th edn. Wadsworth, California

Ekman P (1992) Are there basic emotions? *Psychol Rev* **99**: 550–3

Ellsworth PC, Carlsmith JM (1973) Eye contact and gaze aversion in aggressive encounter. *J Pers Soc Psychol* **33**: 117–22

Hadlow J, Pitts M (1991) The understanding of common health terms by doctors, nurses and patients. *Soc Sci Med* **32**(2): 193–6

Halliday MAK (1978) *Language as Social Semiotic*. Arnold, London

Hymes D (1967) Models of interaction and language and social setting. *J Soc Issues* **23**

Kreps GL, O'Hair D, Clowers Hart M (1995) Communication and health. In: Kreps GL, O'Hair D, eds. *Communication and Health Outcomes*. Hampton Press, Cresskill, New Jersey

Nelson-Jones R (2000) *Practical Counselling and Helping Skills*. 4th edn. Cassell, London

Rogers CR (1980) *A Way of Being*. Houghton Mifflin, Boston

Rozin P, Lowery L, Ebert R (1994) Varieties of disgust faces and the structure of disgust. *J Pers Soc Psychol* **66**: 870–81

Sutherland HJ, Lockwood GA, Tritchler DL *et al* (1991) Communicating probabilistic information to cancer patients: Is there 'noise' on the line? *Soc Sci Med* **32**(6): 725–31

Thompson N (1994) *People Skills: A guide to effective practice in the human service*. Macmillan, Basingstoke

Williams D (1997) *Communication Skills in Practice: A practical guide for health professionals*. Jessica Kingsley, London

Section II:
Application to practice

6

Pregnancy: a time of change and uncertainty

Nearly all women, at some point during their lives, expect to become mothers and will experience pregnancy and childbirth, but relatively few researchers have considered what these life events mean to women. Why do some women enjoy the entire experience, relishing their changing shape and looking forward eagerly to the birth, while others hate the whole nine months? Obviously, the answer to these questions lies in the fact that the experience of pregnancy varies enormously from individual to individual and no two pregnancies are alike (Raphael-Leff, 1991). A host of factors influence how pregnancy will be perceived. These may include among other things: a woman's past history, her psychological coping skills, her socio-economic status, the social support she receives, recent life events and whether the pregnancy is planned or unplanned.

The aim of this chapter is to focus on women's **experience** of pregnancy. This is slightly different from most medically-orientated texts, which consider pregnancy from a biological viewpoint. These accounts of pregnancy tend to reflect the obstetrician's view that pregnancy is abnormal and risky (Schuman and Marteau, 1993) and complications of pregnancy are emphasised.

> *Pregnancy, as a profound physical transformation, is delineated in medical and nursing texts by its physiology and its signs and symptoms, but such explanations do not address the complex and interwoven nature for a woman, of her bodily experience and her sense of changing self.*
>
> (Marck, 1994, p. 90)

Such texts tend to ignore the fact that pregnancy is not only a biological event but also has **cultural** meanings (Oakley, 1980). Inadvertently perhaps, medically-orientated texts de-individualise women and ignore what pregnancy signifies to them. While it is undeniably true that midwives must understand the biological progression of pregnancy and the problems that might arise, a full understanding and an empathetic approach to women in pregnancy and labour, is only possible if the biological, personal and cultural meanings are combined and seen as contributory factors in a woman's experience.

In general, although there is an abundance of professional opinion regarding pregnancy, we do not have access to women's accounts of their experiences (Kaplan, 1992):

> *But what do we hear from women? Where are their voices?... surrounded by others' thoughts on their experiences, few women, it seems, are asked to voice their own.*

(Marck, 1994, p. 82)

This chapter, drawing on feminist-orientated writing, as well as more traditional psychological research, attempts to understand pregnancy as it might be seen from the perspective of women rather than the medical profession. Instead of being the 'object' of medical attention, the woman herself is placed in the foreground, her experiences are valued as important and she is regarded as an 'expert' in terms of her own pregnancy. Her experience of pregnancy is seen as significant and worthy of research in its own right. Such a woman-centred approach accords with the view put forward by the recent *Changing Childbirth* document which clearly states, not only that every woman is an individual and has unique needs, but that:

> *The woman must be the focus of maternity care. She should be able to feel that she is in control of what is happening to her and able to make decisions about her care, based on her needs.*

(DoH, 1993, p. 9)

This approach will be helpful in enabling the midwife to understand that for every woman pregnancy is a unique experience and will encourage her, in her everyday dealings with pregnant women, to 'hear their story'. It is crucial to respond to women as individuals and, by doing so, you will help both to empower them and work with them in a way that is more beneficial to the mother's well being and more satisfying to you as the midwife.

Adjustments to pregnancy

Pregnancy profoundly affects every aspect of a woman's life and she must adapt her behaviour and thinking to enable her to cope with the changes that are occurring within her. In essence, women must come to understand themselves differently during pregnancy. This chapter is structured around the idea that the adaptations that women have to make to pregnancy take place on three different but interrelated dimensions, namely: psychological, behavioural and social.

Psychologically, the pregnant woman has to come to terms with and understand her new role and so for many women, pregnancy may be a time of conflicting emotions. If the pregnancy is long awaited then the response may be one of overwhelming happiness, but even this could be mixed with anxieties about the possibility of medical complications during pregnancy or worries associated with the health of the baby. On the other hand, an unplanned or unwanted pregnancy may be greeted with disappointment and despondency. Whether a woman's reaction is positive or negative, we can be reasonably certain that there will be an emotional response of some sort as she readjusts to her new condition.

A woman who is pregnant may also feel the need to change her **behaviour**. She may try to be more health conscious, eating carefully and resting more than she did before she became pregnant. She may also avoid substances that might harm the unborn child by giving up smoking, and refraining from taking alcohol or drugs.

These areas of change and adaptation are not mutually exclusive, but arc interlinked and effect each other in complex ways. For example, a woman who feels positive about her pregnancy may find the physical changes easy to cope with. On the other hand, a woman who is anxious about the bodily changes that accompany pregnancy may find it difficult to adjust to her increasing weight and changing shape. It is also important to be aware that none of the changes that women make when adjusting to their pregnancy take place in a social vacuum. Later on in the chapter we will consider how the **social and cultural** meaning of pregnancy influences a woman's experience.

Psychological adjustments

During pregnancy women may experience mood swings, memory lapse and heightened emotionality: in addition, women may find themselves turning inward and becoming more introspective as if they need to concentrate on what is happening to them and to their bodies. Although there has been a lot of research on the postpartum, in particular postnatal depression, there has been relatively little work on the psychology of pregnancy. Some studies have been carried out on cognitive failure, anxiety, and coping with loss.

Cognitive failure

Within cultural stereotypes of pregnancy there are various assumptions made about the ways in which women change psychologically. Perhaps one of the dominant ideas is that women become forgetful and absentminded, unable to cope with tasks that previously they had no difficulty with. Such cognitive failure may be explained as:

> *... becoming forgetful, finding it difficult to concentrate or plan, making errors in tasks previously able to accomplish, making verbal slips, doing something at the wrong time.*

(Gross and Pattison, 1995, p. 17)

Women themselves report that they are more likely to experience cognitive failure when pregnant, but although studies have explored this phenomena in the general population, relatively little research has been carried out on pregnant women.

Jarrahi-Zadeh *et al* (1961) studied eighty-six pregnant women who were in their third trimester or had already given birth. These researchers found some reduction in cognitive functioning, as did Poser *et al* (1986). Of the fifty-one women who participated in this study, twenty-one reported cognitive dysfunction of one kind or another, the most common being forgetfulness. A more recent study by Brindle *et al* (1991) also indicates some memory impairment in pregnant women.

Gross and Pattison (1995) studied thirty-one pregnant women throughout their pregnancies, asking them to complete Broadbent's Cognitive Failure Questionnaire every four weeks. The women who participated came from a variety of backgrounds and had different levels of educational achievement, ranging from none at all to degree level. All the subjects were primiparous. A comparison group of similar but non-pregnant women was also recruited. The results of this study indicated that while some women do experience cognitive failure in pregnancy, this was not true for everyone. Women who had experienced pre-menstrual tension before becoming pregnant were more likely to suffer from cognitive failure. They also found higher cognitive failure in the sample around the fourth month of pregnancy that tailed off by the seventh month. There was no relationship between age and cognitive failure.

Summarising the results from these studies it would appear that while cognitive failure does not affect all pregnant women there are a minority for whom it is significant and explanations for why it occurs have been suggested by a number of researchers. Jarrahi-Zadeh *et al* (1961) argue that biological factors were influential, this is supported to some extent by the findings of Gross and Pattison (1995) who noted that women who had experienced pre-menstrual tension were more likely to experience cognitive failure than women who had not. Purvin and Dunn (1987) argued that memory loss could be due to lifestyle changes, such as the restriction of caffeine, but this has not been supported by other studies. Another explanation is that cognitive failure tends to occur generally at any time of life when an individual is experiencing stress and change. As already noted, pregnancy is a time of great change and so this could well be the answer. The study by Gross and Pattison provides a certain degree of support for this explanation, the rise in cognitive failure around the fourth month coincides with clinical visits and potentially stressful tests for fetal abnormalities, while the drop in cognitive failure around the seventh month occurred at the time when most of the women in the sample were giving up work and did not have to cope with so many different demands on their time.

The psychoanalytic school would offer yet another explanation: changes in cognitive functioning occur because a woman becomes inward looking during her pregnancy as she reflects on the processes that are going on within her body. This absorbs her whole being and there is little mental capacity left over for the more mundane aspects of everyday life. Winnicott (1958) calls this, 'primary mental pre-occupation'.

Rubin (1961) believes that there is much cognitive work that needs to be done during pregnancy as the mother adjusts to her changing role and this is manifested in less rational, but more intuitive thinking. Cognitive failure is an inappropriate term as during pregnancy cognitive activity is intense as women mentally prepare themselves for motherhood. This involves modelling maternal behaviour (role-play), fantasising about becoming a mother (where the role-play becomes internalised), and finally coming to a conclusion about what kind of a mother she will be (Mercer, 1995).

Of course there are many criticisms that could be levelled at these explanations, the principal one being that they are largely theoretical and not supported by experimental evidence. While there is no doubt that this is a major difficulty, psychoanalytic explanations frequently provide helpful insights into behaviour and cannot simply be dismissed because they are seen as being 'unscientific'. We will consider the psychoanalytic ideas about the psychological changes of pregnancy in more detail later in the chapter.

Given that the studies that have been carried out on cognitive failure are relatively few in number and have not studied large samples of women, it is probably premature to attempt to draw firm conclusions about the causes of cognitive failure in pregnancy. What is clear is that some women are affected and this could cause additional difficulties particularly for those who have demanding jobs to cope with for the duration of the pregnancy.

Anxiety

As pregnancy is a time of change and uncertainty, it is not unreasonable to assume that women will experience increased levels of anxiety during this period of their lives. There are many potential difficulties that a woman might worry about in terms of her own health or that of her unborn baby. Antenatal screening has to be coped with and may be particularly stressful. In later pregnancy women may feel concerned about labour and whether they will be able to control the pain, some women may even feel anxious about motherhood and wonder if they will be able to manage after the birth. Although anxiety during pregnancy is something that appears to be a logical consequence of pregnancy itself, research findings about the extent and intensity of anxiety during the antenatal period have not always been consistent and it remains unclear whether raised levels of anxiety are a symptom of pregnancy or not. Research that has focused on anxiety relating to antenatal screening procedures and other *specific* stressors have found these to be associated with increased levels of anxiety.

In a large study of nearly 1000 Indian women, Singh and Saxena (1991) found that the 691 pregnant women in their sample experienced more anxiety than the control group. Anxiety began in the second month of pregnancy as soon as the women knew that they were pregnant and continued to rise up to the fifth month. There was a slight decrease in anxiety in the sixth and seventh months, and another increase in the eighth and ninth months as pregnancy came to an end. Levels of anxiety decreased markedly once the baby had been born and continued to decrease up until six months after the birth. This study used a simple state anxiety questionnaire and so gives no indication as to what the women in the study were anxious about.

Studies in Europe and the USA do not appear to have demonstrated the same general increase in anxiety throughout pregnancy that Singh and Saxena found. There could be several reasons for this. There will inevitably be cultural differences in the way women approach pregnancy and it is possible that for Indian women, there is more fear surrounding pregnancy than for Western women. This could be due to greater knowledge about pregnancy and childbirth in the more industrialised cultures engendering more confidence about the whole process. Another explanation could be that the infant and maternal mortality rate is high in India and women might reasonably be expected to be anxious about the outcome of their pregnancy.

Studies that have looked at specific stressors in pregnancy have found raised levels of anxiety in a number of situations. A study of Swedish women (Welles-Nystrom and de Chateau, 1987) found that older first time mothers (30–39 years) showed a tendency to be more anxious than a younger group of primigravida (20–29 years). Although these results appear to accord with common sense; one might expect older women to be more anxious because of the perceived increased risk of pregnancy in older women, caution needs to be exercised in interpreting the findings. The sample was relatively small with only fifty participants and not all of the older mothers showed raised levels of anxiety.

As *Table 6.1* indicates, eleven of the twenty-six older mothers showed anxiety compared to six of the twenty-seven younger mothers. Although this result was significant and demonstrated that the proportion of older mothers who were anxious was greater than the proportion of younger women experiencing anxiety, it still left fifteen of the older group who did not appear to exhibit anxiety. Using these results it would be misguided for the midwife to make the assumption that all older primigravida will show raised levels of anxiety.

Table 6.1: Women experiencing raised levels of anxiety in pregnancy (Welles-Nystrom, de Chateau, 1987)

Characteristics	Group 1 age 20–29 (n=27)	Group 2 age 30–39 (n=26)
Anxious	6	11
Not anxious	21	15

Almost certainly, experience of previous miscarriage or stillbirth will lead to raised levels of anxiety in subsequent pregnancies. In an in-depth analysis of ten women who had experienced stillbirth, Lever Hense (1994) found that anxiety was common. Women reported feeling worried about the pregnancy and labour, and found that they associated labour with death rather than life. This is discussed more fully in *Chapter 10*.

A lot of attention has been paid to the effects of antenatal screening procedures on levels of anxiety and have demonstrated that such procedures do raise anxiety, although this is only temporary. Michelacci *et al* (1988) looking at a group of Italian women found that:

> ... *psychological reactions to ultrasound examination are intense and varied.*

> (p. 3)

These researchers studied the same women on three occasions and found high anxiety levels each time; however, raised levels of anxiety preceding ultrasound quickly disappeared after the successful completion of the scan. Interestingly, they also found raised levels of other psychological reactions such as depression, somatic symptoms and hostility. In this paper the authors raise the question of whether the anxiety induced by screening outweighs the benefits in a normal pregnancy.

On the other hand, Marteau *et al* (1988) found that in women who were perceived to be 'at risk' for fetal abnormalities, screening procedures could serve to reduce anxiety in the long term. Women who had undergone amniocentesis to detect Down's syndrome or had been screened for neural tube defect showed less anxiety in the third trimester of pregnancy, presumably because they were secure in the knowledge that their baby was healthy. The authors of this paper rightly point out that every woman will perceive any screening procedure in a way that is individual to her. For some, it will be seen positively as a chance to check that things are normal, while for others it will be seen as threatening.

> *For some women, such as those who know that they are at risk of producing a child with a congenital abnormality... the chance to undergo prenatal diagnostic testing may provide a relief, a negative result serving to reassure them throughout the rest of their pregnancy. For women who*

enter pregnancy unaware of any raised risk... the offer of prenatal diagnostic testing may be a challenge to their pregnancy.

(Marteau *et al*, 1988, p. 8)

Some researchers have considered the effects that raised levels of anxiety might have on the fetus. Rossi *et al* (1989) demonstrated that fetal motor activity lasted longer in women undergoing amniocentesis than in a control group who were having a routine ultrasound scan. Although the fetus appeared more active in women awaiting amniocentesis, there were no significant differences in smaller movements such as moving the hand towards the face or movement of the limbs or in overall number of movements in the ten-minute observation period. In the introduction to their paper these authors discuss a number of studies which claim to have shown a relationship between maternal anxiety and higher incidences of obstetric complications and 'neonatal suffering', but it is not made clear how such a brief period of anxiety during antenatal screening could have long term consequences for the unborn child, or how anxiety *per se* could translate into neonatal suffering or obstetric complications. Rossi *et al* give no indication of the mechanism by which these problems could occur. It seems to me that there is every chance that women who are extremely anxious during pregnancy have other things going on in their lives that could contribute to the difficulties they and their babies might experience. It is unlikely that anxiety is the only contributory factor.

Van den Bergh (1990) has also noted that maternal anxiety is linked with more intense fetal movements, and this author quotes several studies that have demonstrated that, 'mothers under severe emotional stress tend to have hyperactive foetuses' (Van den Bergh, 1990). However, unlike the previous researchers Van den Bergh is more cautious about the conclusions he draws from his findings. Although the results of thirty women experiencing anxiety during pregnancy demonstrate that both fetal movements and the behaviour of the neonate are affected, Van den Bergh points out that the correlations are small and 'much of the variance remains unexplained' (p. 127).

So, where does all of this leave us? Can we conclude that anxiety in pregnancy is common or that it has an adverse effect on the fetus and neonate? It seems that the assumption that pregnant women will be overly anxious is not really borne out by the research that has been done in the field. Undoubtedly some women do become anxious

(Lever Hense, 1994) and experience moments of extreme stress during screening procedures, but the majority of women whose pregnancies are normal and going well, do not appear to experience anxiety to a greater degree than other members of the population. Similarly, the evidence to date does appear to demonstrate that anxiety has some effect on the fetus, making it more active in utero. However, it is not possible to conclude that anxiety causes this. Just like the fictitious experiment on sleep described in *Chapter 1*, there are too many variables that could be influencing the results that have not been accounted for.

From the point of view of the midwife, this uncertainty may be confusing. What can we conclude — are pregnant woman anxious or not? The research that we have looked at provides some evidence for greater levels of anxiety during pregnancy but it does not allow us to generalise to all pregnant women and all we can really say is that some women will experience anxiety during pregnancy, while others will not. Although this may seem unsatisfactory, there is something to be gained from the findings. Such research highlights two points that are relevant for midwifery practice. Firstly, that anxiety during pregnancy does occur quite commonly, particularly during screening and at other times when a woman is aware of potential health problems in her unborn child. Secondly, that every woman's reaction to pregnancy and screening is different, underlining both the danger of making broad generalisations about pregnant women and the importance of responding to each woman as an individual who will have her own idiosyncratic way of dealing with her pregnancy.

Experience of loss

Any life change, however positive, involves loss, and pregnancy is no exception. In addition to dealing with anxiety and cognitive failure, women may also have to come to terms with a sense of loss for what has changed and will never be the same again.

> ... *all pregnancy involves loss. For the woman having a child entails loss of unquestioned singleness in her body, loss of her physical well-being, loss of her figure, her carefree social life, postponement of career or occupation...*
>
> (Raphael-Leff, 1991, p. 16)

Rubin (1984) argues that women have to engage in grief work during pregnancy, this involves 'relinquishing any role or identity that is incompatible with the forthcoming maternal role. Giving up current life-style also involves grief work' (quoted in Mercer, 1995, p. 59).

Such negative thoughts do not sit easily with the rather rosy cultural stereotypes of pregnancy that are reflected everywhere in society and this mismatch between individual experience and societal expectations frequently makes it difficult for women to acknowledge their conflicting feelings. Nevertheless, women may well feel sad about some of the changes that pregnancy brings. Many women report that they feel their girlhood has come to an end once they become pregnant. Now they really are grown-ups with adult responsibilities that will remain with them for the rest of their lives.

Over several years of talking about the experience of loss in pregnancy with midwifery students I have asked them to imagine what losses women may have to confront during pregnancy. The ideas that students have come up with are shown in *Table 6.2*. I am sure that you can think of others that you may wish to add to the list. My aim is not so much to attempt to enumerate every loss that a woman might experience but simply to raise the issue of

Table 6.2: Losses in pregnancy
Identity/self-concept
Independence
Individuality
Career
Control
Body image
Sexuality
Sexual attractiveness
Girlhood
Valued activities
Pregnancy (miscarriage)

coping with loss in pregnancy and discuss the general principle of a woman's need to come to terms with this.

One important aspect of loss to note is that they rarely come alone, one thing influences another and there is a cascade effect. Consider a woman who becomes a widow, not only does she lose her partner's company, but she may also lose financial security. This may mean that she has to give up certain valued activities. She might also feel that she has lost her identity and status in society. She might even lose her home and valued friendships. As with this example, so it is in pregnancy too.

If we look at pregnancy from a purely biological perspective then it can be regarded as normal and natural; women should be able to adapt to it easily and with no psychological ill effects, but as I have already argued, pregnancy is not only a biological event. It takes place within a complex cultural setting (Oakley, 1980); this has many implications for women and effects every detail of their life. If a woman has a career then she may feel or will be expected to put it on hold while she has her children. This could mean that she will never achieve the standing in her professional life that she would have done had she not had children. If much of her identity is tied up with her work then she will experience loss of identity too.

She may lose a sense of independence and individuality because, unlike her partner, she has to learn to share her body with another individual, it is no longer her own. It becomes the receptacle for another life and in another sense becomes the property of the medical profession. She must endure tests and examinations often of a personal nature, she must be careful about what she eats and what she does, not just for her own health and well being but for the sake of the baby. It is hardly surprising that some women describe pregnancy as a kind of invasion of their body.

Her body is changing rapidly too; this may lead to a feeling that she is losing control. The baby grows despite her, her breasts change and she puts on weight. The body she has known well now responds differently to food, she may feel sick and unwell. If body image has been an important part of a woman's self-concept then loss of her figure might be very challenging and require a major readjustment. Her changing body image may influence her sexuality too, she may feel more or less sexually attractive or feel that her carefree sexual life has come to an end. Society invests so much in the ideal of the slim non-pregnant, sexually available female body and the state of pregnancy runs counter to this entirely. The non-pregnant body is OK, the pregnant one is not and inevitably women's feelings about themselves when pregnant are influenced by this discourse. (It always strikes me as strange that in almost every paper and magazine you open there are images of naked breasts, however, when breasts are depicted being used for their real purpose of feeding infants there is public revulsion.)

Valued activities might come to an end for all kinds of reasons. The development of the pregnancy might prevent certain kinds of active sports where an injury could prove damaging to the baby. Loss of income through giving up work could mean that, financially, certain activities are impossible. A woman may even look forward to the time when the baby is born and grieve for activities that used to be enjoyed but will be impossible with a small baby in tow, such as shopping for clothes or going to the cinema.

Of course, the most significant loss of all is the loss of the pregnancy through miscarriage or stillbirth. I intend to leave the discussion of this to the chapter that deals with loss and bereavement, where I consider the effect of miscarriage, stillbirth and neonatal death. I do this because many of the losses that we have discussed so far are more or less reversible. Women do get their figures back, they are able to pick up valued activities again, and it is often helpful for women to be reassured about this. However, loss involving a death of some kind is not reversible and even though a woman becomes pregnant again, it is not the same; the lost baby can never be replaced.

Depression

A great deal of research has been carried out on postnatal depression, but depression during pregnancy is common too and some researchers have argued that postnatal depression is simply an extension of depression experienced antenatally. Although hormonal explanations for depression during the reproductive period have been sought, there has been little consensus in the literature and a biological cause still eludes researchers. If, as I have suggested above, many women experience a sense of loss during pregnancy and need to engage in what Rubin calls grief work, then it would be reasonable to expect these women to feel depressed too. Loss of any kind is usually accompanied by grief (Parkes, 1976) and this would be as true in pregnancy as in any other stage of life. A full discussion of depression in pregnancy and the puerperium can be found in *Chapter 9*.

Psychological change in pregnancy: the psycho-analytical viewpoint

It would take several volumes to give a full account of the various psychoanalytic writers who have put forward theories to explain what they believe is happening to women as they go through pregnancy, so only a brief account is given here to give a 'feel' for this approach. A fuller description can be found in Raphael-Leff and Perelberg (1997).

As already indicated, the psychoanalytic approach to pregnancy is qualitatively different from mainstream psychological literature. The methods of analysis are not experimental, the evidence comes mainly from psychotherapeutic work. Consequently, with pregnant women there is more emphasis on internal and emotional processes and less on the effects of culture and environment. Although these methods have been widely criticised for being unscientific, in general, psychoanalytically-orientated writers have paid more attention to women's *experiences* of pregnancy than other psychologists.

As we saw in the introductory chapter, Freud, the founding father of psychoanalytic theory, believed that human sexuality was fundamental to human experience. Although other writers have challenged Freud's ideas about the centrality of sexuality in the development of the psyche, it is still the case that almost all psychoanalytic theory believes this aspect of the individual to be a fundamental driving force in behaviour. This inevitably has an impact on pregnancy and childbirth, these being the logical conclusion of (hetero)sexual activity.

The logic behind the relationship between sexuality and human behaviour is as follows: at the most basic level, sexuality is bio-logically driven. We have little control over our sexual development; puberty begins according to some inner biological clock, as does the menopause. Without artificial means we cannot control when we ovulate. This is also true of pregnancy, although modern women have the ability to control whether they become pregnant or not, after conception biology takes over. Freud believed that the development of our sexual selves underpinned many other aspects of personality development. As pregnancy is the natural endpoint of sexual development in women, it follows that pregnancy must be a highly significant event in life, and is closely related to inner experience of herself. Because of its links with sexual behaviour, a woman's experience of pregnancy is likely to link back to previous aspects of sexual development and reawaken issues from childhood that have not yet been resolved.

Freud himself took a rather negative view of female sexuality, seeing female development as inferior to the development of the male. He believed that women suffered from penis envy and that this could only be resolved by becoming pregnant and bearing a (preferably male) child. Later writers such as Deutsh, Horney, Klein and Anna Freud (Sayers, 1991) have taken a more positive view of female sexuality and motherhood and have emphasised the significance of a woman's capacity to mother a child and breast-feed. From a modern perspective, it seems likely that the negative view Freud took of women's sexuality was indeed a reflection of the time in which he lived, when women were very much restricted and might justifiably envy men the freedom that possession of a penis gave them.

More recent psychoanalytic theorists have broadened our view of pregnancy and motherhood. This new approach to psychoanalytic thought began during the 1920s and 1930s when women psychoanalysts began to question Freud's phallo-centric approach to human development. Object relations theory, which highlights the theoretical and clinical significance of the infant-mother relationship, was the result of this reorientation in thinking. This work has its own particular flavour, concentrating on the mother's bond with the fetus and the ways in which she has to accommodate herself to her changing status. The transition from being someone's daughter to becoming a mother herself requires the formation of a new identity, the mother-to-be might harbour all kinds of fantasies about her unborn baby, ranging from the sex of the baby to the hopes and fears that she may hold for his or her future. Such fantasies are thought to be an important part of the cognitive work that all women engage in as they assume the role of 'mother' (Rubin, 1961). According to Raphael-Leff (1991), women might feel more connected to humanity once they are pregnant, seeing themselves as part of a continuing line of mothers from generation to generation.

Pregnancy, like many other major changes in life, has the ability to reawaken old and deep issues, childhood conflicts may surface again and women may well need to re-evaluate both themselves and their relationships with parents and partners.

What I find markedly apparent during pregnancy is an involuntary 'permeability' a loosening of internal barriers between levels of consciousness and within memory. Thoughts, feelings and fantasies which are usually subliminal suddenly seep into consciousness and must either be attended to or effortfully kept at bay.

(Raphael-Leff, 1991, p. 49)

Several writers assume that the wish to be or become pregnant is not random, but is motivated by deep inner needs which may also date back to early, unresolved childhood issues that may now be dealt with as the woman goes through pregnancy.

There are many criticisms of psychoanalytic theory, by its very nature, it is extremely difficult to prove or disprove the concepts contained therein. Theories are often developed from clinical work done with only a small number of clients and many would argue that these are people with 'problems' who are not representative of the population at large. Because of these limitations, some more experimentally-orientated psychologists would dismiss the ideas entirely.

While I have some sympathy with these criticisms, it is my feeling that we cannot simply discard psychoanalytic theory. There are at least two reasons for this. Firstly, psychoanalytic theory has had a major impact on modern thinking about human motivation and we cannot escape from it. Terms that derive from psychoanalytic theory, such as 'Freudian slip', the unconscious, defence mechanisms and regression are now part of our everyday language. We believe that our past is important and that it has played a role in whom we are today. We believe that the mother/infant relationship is fundamental to development. We think sexuality is a significant part of our behaviour. All of these ideas originate from psychoanalytic theory and have become incorporated into the way in which we conceptualise behaviour so that to some extent we all make sense of others and ourselves from a psychoanalytic perspective. This will be true of many pregnant women with whom you are working, as well as you yourself. This alone is not a sufficient reason to accept psychoanalytic theory. Of far more importance is the fact that it can be a useful tool in helping us to develop a deeper understanding of human behaviour. Many of the concepts enable us to gain a greater awareness of the individual and to explain behaviour that may, on the surface, appear to be irrational. This can help us to deal with people more sensitively and not to dismiss anxieties and fears, as well as aggressive behaviour, out of hand. Even if we do not wholeheartedly subscribe to every aspect of psychoanalytic theory, we cannot deny that such explanations have a richness and depth and certainly give us insight into the human condition.

Having very briefly outlined some of the ideas, I will leave you to make up your own mind and perhaps do some more reading around the subject (a good introduction is edited by Raphael-Leff and Perelberg, 1997). My experience with students' responses to the approach is that there is no middle ground; you either find it fascinating and want to learn more, or dismiss it totally. Of course, if you do tend towards the latter view, it means that you find the whole thing too threatening and are using defence mechanisms to protect yourself from dealing with such issues! Whichever way you jump, it is certainly an approach that must be considered.

Adjustments in behaviour

It is inevitable that during pregnancy a woman's behaviour has to change. Initially, in the first trimester, tiredness and nausea may mean that she has to rest more and be careful about the food she eats. Most women report feeling healthy and active during the second trimester, but in the third trimester increase in size will once again mean that she will have to accommodate her behaviour to her physical state and she may feel tired, breathless and too bulky to engage in much physical activity.

To a large extent the changes in behaviour that I have just described are involuntary, brought about because of the physical demands of the pregnancy, but other adjustments in behaviour could be due to a conscious decision to engage in health-related behaviour for the duration of the pregnancy. It is now well documented that smoking, drinking alcohol and taking drugs have negative consequences for the development of the fetus and many women are prepared to refrain from these activities until after the baby is born. They may also be more careful about their food and caffeine intake and take vitamin supplements such as folic acid. Attendance at antenatal classes and checks may also be regarded as a way of safeguarding the health of herself and her baby.

As all of these behaviours are regarded by health professionals as a way of maintaining maternal and fetal health; there has been a concern to encourage pregnant women to change their behaviour in positive ways. The concept of locus of control has been useful in helping psychologists to understand why some people are more prepared to engage in behaviours that will have a positive impact on their health than others. The idea was originally developed by Rotter in 1954. He:

> *... made the distinction between internal and external locus of control orientations: 'internals' are seen to believe that events are a consequence of their own actions and thereby under personal control, whereas 'externals' are seen to believe that events are unrelated to their actions and thereby determined by factors beyond their personal control.*

(Norman and Bennett, 1996, p. 63)

Rotter's theory suggests that people with an internal locus of control believe that they have the ability to influence the things that happen to them in their lives, while those with an external locus of control believe that they have little or no ability to affect what happens to them. Although Rotter did not apply his ideas specifically to health-related behaviours, Strickland (1978) argued that people who have an internal locus of control are more likely to believe that they can control their health and well being by behaving in ways that are likely to benefit them, while those who have an external locus of control think that whatever they do, it will have little or no effect on the outcome.

Rotter produced a scale to measure whether people were internals or externals and initially, this was used to measure health behaviours. However, this general scale was inadequate and a more specific one, the Multidimensional Health Locus of Control Scale (MHLC) was developed which had the advantage of distinguishing between those externals who believed that control was held by powerful others and those who believed in chance or fate (Wallston *et al*, 1978).

Relating this idea to the pregnant woman, the theory would predict that those with an internal locus of control would take an active part in their pregnancy, would seek out information about it and would attempt to engage in behaviours that would be likely to have positive benefits. Women with an external locus of control who believed in the power of chance or fate, would be inclined to think that their health was out of their control and would be less likely to engage in beneficial health-related activities. A woman with an external locus of control, who believed in the influence of powerful others, may be more willing to put her trust in doctors and midwives and do whatever they tell her. Wallston (1992) has argued that this orientation could be effective for people when they are ill and for some pregnant women, it could have some positive benefits too.

Attempts to use the MHLC scale on pregnant women were not successful because the questions were not specific enough. This led Labs and Wurtele (1986) to develop a scale called the Fetal-Health Locus of Control Scale (FHLC), which is designed to measure whether a woman's belief in her ability to influence the health of her unborn child will have an impact on her behaviour during pregnancy. Based on the MHLC, the FHLC contains:

> *An internal dimension measuring a woman's belief that she is directly responsible for the health of her unborn child (**Internal**) and two external dimensions assessing*

*beliefs that health professionals (**Powerful others**) and
chance factors (**Chance**) determine the newborn's health.*

(Labs and Wurtele, 1986, p. 817, author's emphasis)

Their sample consisted of sixty-three pregnant women and they
found that internals were more likely to refrain from smoking during
pregnancy and consume less caffeine. These women were also more
likely to state their intention of participating in the antenatal classes.
Tinsley *et al* (1993) using a different scale called the Pregnancy
Belief Scale, which like other health locus of control scales measured
internality, chance externality and powerful others externality, found
that women who believed that they could influence their birth outcomes were likely to take better care of themselves during
pregnancy. This in turn was related to a better birth outcome. Unlike
the study of Labs and Wurtele, Tinsley *et al* did not rely on self-
reports of compliance to health-related behaviour, but measured this
from the medical reports of physicians. Their findings did not account
for all the variance which led them to the more tentative conclusion
that:

*Pregnancy related health locus of control beliefs appear
to be one of many factors that relate to and may contribute
to individual differences in women's prenatal health and
birth outcomes.*

(Tinsley *et al*, 1993, p. 101)

The results of these studies appear to give the clear message that
having an internal locus of control is of positive benefit to the
individual: such women will engage in behaviours that are likely to
lead to a beneficial outcome for their own health and the health of the
unborn child. Research has also shown that there may be an occasion
when having an external (powerful others) locus of control is
preferable. Reisch and Tinsley (1994) studied a group of impoverished
American women with low education levels and found that an
external locus of control was a better predictor of a number of
prenatal visits and birth outcome. The authors argued that when
people are in situations where there really is no hope of control over
the environment, externals with a belief in powerful others are better
adapted to cope. Internals who live in situations where they have no
hope of taking control constantly experience failure.

In other circumstances too, internals may not fare so well. They
may be less willing to conform to the demands of the midwife or

obstetrician and may feel unable to hand control over to other people, which is often essential in complicated labours. This may make them appear 'difficult' to health professionals who may then be less sympathetic. By comparison, externals who believe in powerful others, may appear much easier to deal with as they are more likely to put their trust in the doctor or midwife and do as they are told.

The most potentially difficult individuals in terms of conformity to health behaviours are those who have an external locus of control, but who believe in fate. This group seem the least likely to engage in positive behaviours to enhance their own health or the health of the baby.

Of course, much of this is speculation and more research on locus of control and pregnancy needs to be carried out. As Tinsley *et al* (1993) pointed out, there is a great deal of variation in health-related behaviour that remains unaccounted for. Ethnic background, social class (Rutter, Quine and Hayward, 1988), previous obstetric history (Bielawska-Batorowicz, 1993), marital satisfaction (Zimmermann-Tansella *et al*, 1994), availability of transport may all influence a woman's preparedness to engage in behaviour that will enhance her health during pregnancy.

An alternative way of making sense of whether people engage in health-related behaviours, which incorporates some of these issues is the health belief model. This model recognises that demographic variables such as class, gender and age, as well as psychological characteristics like personality and peer group pressure have an impact on behaviour. In addition, an individual's perception of their susceptibility to an illness and its severity will influence health behaviours — susceptibility and severity is balanced against perceived benefits and barriers to the health behaviour. Overlying all of this is the individuals' motivation to remain healthy.

Perhaps this model is best understood with an example. An extremely overweight woman might be told that she needs to lose weight because of the danger to her health. Whether she does so will depend on her overall motivation, on whether she thinks she is likely to become ill (susceptibility) and how bad she believes the illness is likely to be (severity). In addition, she will need to believe that the benefits to be gained from losing weight outweigh (no pun intended) the costs of dieting, and she will have to overcome barriers to this change in behaviour. Demographic variables and her own psychological characteristics will also contribute to her success or failure at losing weight.

In some ways, the health belief model is perhaps a better predictor of women's health behaviour during pregnancy than the locus of control model, although at times both may need to be employed to understand why an individual finds it difficult to change or to motivate a person to make changes that would benefit both their own and their baby's health.

Social and cultural influences

Although pregnancy and childbirth are fundamentally biological events, they are also significant social happenings, which have an impact not only on the woman herself but on the social group to which she belongs. When a baby is born everyone in the immediate social circle has to make adjustments to incorporate this new group member. Oakley expresses this beautifully:

> *Childbirth stands uncomfortably at the junction of the two worlds of nature and culture. Like death and disease it is a biological event, but the defining feature of biological events in human life is their social character. The way people are born and die.... cannot be explained purely on the basis of knowledge about the biological functioning of the human organism. Bodies function in a social world....*

> (Oakley, 1980, p. 7)

When looking at the social influences that have an impact on a woman's experience of pregnancy we can see the individual as being part of a small social network that makes up the group of people with whom she interacts on a daily basis. This group will be made up of family, friends, work colleagues etc. However, this group is itself part of a wider culture which will have an impact on how women make sense of pregnancy, childbirth and motherhood. We could regard the pregnant woman as existing within three concentric circles (*Figure 6.1*). The inner circle represents herself; the second circle represents her personal social sphere; and the outer circle consists of the wider society in which she lives. All will influence her and have an impact on her experience of pregnancy.

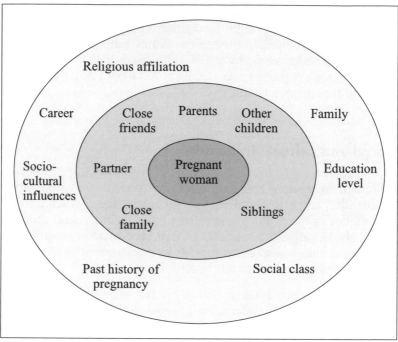

Figure 6.1: Social and cultural influences on the pregnant woman

As we have seen in previous chapters, the social world in which we live subtly influences our behaviour and affects every aspect of our daily lives. Partners may be more or less supportive. Socioeconomic factors might make a pregnancy easier or more difficult to cope with. A woman may be relatively socially isolated, or may be surrounded by loving and helpful family and friends. Social norms will have an impact too, so although pregnancy within a stable relationship is regarded positively, single parenthood, teenage pregnancy or pregnancy in older women has other connotations. This means that an individual may be torn between her own feelings about her pregnancy and societal expectations. A single woman may be delighted to learn of her pregnancy but its social unacceptability could mean that she does not get the same support that a married woman or a woman in a stable relationship would receive and she might be subjected to the prejudiced attitudes of others.

In addition to this, in all cultures there are many social discourses surrounding pregnancy and motherhood that also have an impact on how women experience these events (Phoenix and Woollett, 1991; Glenn, 1994). In Western industrialised societies, one of the most dominant discourses is that pregnancy is 'natural'; something that women 'do' and they are expected to take to it like ducks to water. Those women who do not enjoy pregnancy and motherhood or choose not to become mothers at all, are seen as being odd and unusual if not actually mad. This discourse subtly influences women making it very difficult for them to voice any negative feelings that they may have about pregnancy and motherhood.

Just to complicate matters, there are other common discourses that are contradictory to this. For example, although pregnancy is seen as 'natural' — the fulfilment of what being a woman means — it is also pathologised and women are regarded as needing special, medical care during the nine months of pregnancy. This can lead to confusion on the part of many women. They feel that they cannot trust their own bodies and become fearful and uncertain about their responses to pregnancy.

Another common discourse impacts on how women perceive and experience their bodies during pregnancy. One does not have to look very far to realise that the main (perhaps only) positive image of femininity that we see in Western society is of the young, slim, sexually available woman. Slimming clubs, slimming products, magazines and the media all graphically demonstrate the truth of this. This does not sit well with pregnancy, as during this time the 'perfect' body shape is impossible to achieve. Inevitably, this may have an impact on how women feel about their bodies during pregnancy (Sumner *et al*, 1993). Research indicates that pregnant women are more negative about their bodies than non-pregnant women (Ruggieri *et al*, 1979) and feel less attractive than either non-pregnant or the 'ideal' woman (Moore 1978). Strang and Sullivan (1985) found that women were more positive about their bodies before pregnancy, but felt happier about their bodies post-partum than during pregnancy.

Shuzman (1987) found that although initially most women welcome signs of pregnancy, later on these feelings become less positive. Tanner (1969) suggests that this negativity is to do with a woman's increasing bulk, but social and cultural dimensions must also play a part. We have few positive images of pregnancy that we can draw on. Although pictures of naked women appear everywhere, the few photographs of naked pregnant women that have been published have caused an outcry (remember Demi Moore?). All of which is strange when one considers that pregnancy is the inevitable end-point of feminine sexuality. The mixed message we receive is that, as a woman, you must be young and sexually available, but then become unattractive once pregnant. There is some recent evidence to suggest that at a time in their lives when women are most vulnerable they are at a greater risk of domestic violence (Mezey and Bewley, 1997), another example of societies 'double standard' regarding women and pregnancy.

Some feminist writers such as Jane Ussher and Paula Nicolson have argued strongly that the mixed messages women receive regarding pregnancy and motherhood can lead to feelings of uncertainty and even depression. They suggest that women just cannot win. They are destined to become mothers, but are only considered sexually attractive before pregnancy and motherhood, once they are mothers they are expected to be 'naturals' but are bombarded with advice and literature from so-called 'professionals'. If they don't like motherhood, then they are considered abnormal in some way. Feminist writers believe that all this serves men's needs very efficiently and works effectively to keep women in their place in a patriarchal society. We will return to this argument and discuss it in more detail, when we consider postnatal depression in *Chapter 9*.

Social support in pregnancy

I have argued throughout this chapter that pregnancy is a time of transition and change for women. It is a period in their lives, when everything is in a state of flux. Women might find themselves reassessing their life situation and reinventing their roles — they are no longer single individuals answerable only to themselves, but are now responsible for the health and well being of another life. At this time women need greater levels of social support and research indicates that social support can be beneficial, not only to the woman herself, but to her children too.

Rhoades (1989) asked eighty-six first-time mothers to identify who was most supportive during the transition to motherhood. All the women in this sample were married (unmarried women were excluded) and 77% stated that their partners offered the most support. These participants appeared to adjust more easily to motherhood than individuals who identified either support groups of friends as being most supportive. This study reflects a general assumption in the literature that most pregnant women will be married, and that this will be the most influential relationship in their lives. As Zimmermann-Tansella *et al* argue:

A satisfactory marital relationship becomes particularly important during pregnancy because of the womens' major psychological vulnerability in this period. Pregnant women with positive marital relationships have the least disturbed reactions (to pregnancy), while marital dissatisfaction is associated with depression and heightened diffuse anxiety in late pregnancy.

(1994, p. 559)

The study carried out by Zimmermann-Tansella *et al* used a group of fifty-four Italian women. They were all first time mothers and all married. The researchers administered two questionnaires; the General Health Questionnaire (GHQ) and the Ryle Marital Patterns Test (RMPT) to both partners. They found that women who felt that they received high levels of affection from their partners reported lower levels of symptoms of anxiety and insomnia than other women. They also noted that women who perceived high levels of care from their husbands reported more symptoms, while women suffering from depression were more likely to report that they received low levels of affection from their husband.

Although the two studies that have been discussed indicate that there is some kind of relationship between support in pregnancy and general satisfaction, it is difficult to draw firm conclusions from the results. To begin with, the sample sizes were relatively small and could not be considered as representative of the population in general. In both studies the women were from higher than average socioeconomic groups and were more highly educated. In addition, data generated from questionnaires is limited and can only give broad indications of the complexity of relationships and almost no indication of direction or causality. For example, although the study by Zimmerman-Tansella *et al* highlights a relationship between depression and perceived low levels of affection we have no way of knowing whether the low levels of affection caused the woman to become depressed, or whether the depression made the woman feel as if she was not getting enough affection from her partner. The results do not help us to understand what women 'need' in terms of support during pregnancy.

A further criticism is that by using only married women neither study reflects the growing trend in society of women who are not married having children. Although many unmarried women do have long-term partners who provide the same kind of support as a husband might be expected to do, many single women are now becoming pregnant. Who do they go to for support?

A longitudinal study carried out in Britain by Ann Oakley *et al* (1996) clearly demonstrates how important social support in pregnancy can be for women, and how this support does not necessarily need to come from family or friends. Oakley's study began in 1986 and used a large sample of 509 women. To participate, women had to be booking in before twenty-four weeks' gestation with a singleton pregnancy, be English speaking and have a previous history of at least one low birth weight baby (<2500g). The low birth weight indicated that these women might be considered 'at risk' in some way and, in general, the sample was socially disadvantaged. The women were divided into two groups, 255 receiving 'social intervention' in addition to antenatal care and 254 receiving only normal antenatal care.

Four research midwives were employed to provide the additional social support, which consisted of home visits and twenty-four-hour contact with the research midwife. During the visits, the midwife collected data using semi-structured interview schedules, provided a listening ear, gave practical advice and referred women to other health and social service professionals if needed. The majority of visits were made during pregnancy with one brief postnatal visit.

Although the intervention was relatively simple, results were astonishing. Women were followed up in the postnatal period using medical case notes and a postal questionnaire. These indicated that:

> *There were fewer very low birth weight babies, antenatal hospital admissions, non-spontaneous labours and deliveries in the intervention group. Intervention group babies required less intensive and neonatal care and had better health in the early weeks, according to their mothers. The physical and psychosocial health of the intervention mothers was also better, and their partners were reported as being more helpful in the home.*

(Oakley, 1996, p. 8)

The intervention group was still reporting positive results one year after the birth; and at a seven-year follow-up study (47% of the original sample responded) continued to show benefits to both mothers and their children in terms of physical health and psycho-social outcomes. (Oakley *et al*, 1996). It is incredible to reflect that a simple programme of visits from a health professional could have such long-term advantages even seven years after the original study. These results are extremely positive and have wide-ranging implications; not only do they demonstrate the enormous benefit that can be gained from a relatively straightforward intervention programme in terms of physical and psychological health, they also indicate the central role that can be played by the midwife in helping women deal with pregnancy and the postpartum.

Cultural diversity

In this section on social and cultural influences on pregnancy, I have discussed only Western industrialised societies. Although within this chapter we have considered studies from Greece, India, Denmark and Holland as well as Britain and the US, this is a narrow view. Every culture exerts different influences upon women's experiences of pregnancy and has different customs and practices that women may find more or less helpful in coping with pregnancy and we can often learn a lot from the practices of other groups (Kitzinger, 1989). It would take another book and I would need to become an anthropologist to consider the customs and practices of all cultures. However, the importance of taking into account cultural differences and responding to them appropriately cannot be overemphasised. If you find yourself working with women from other cultures or religions, you should undoubtedly attempt to find out as much as possible about attitudes to pregnancy within that culture and reflect this in your midwifery practice, a good account can be found in Katbamna (2000).

Implications for the midwife

The emphasis throughout this chapter has been on the idea that every pregnancy is unique and no two pregnancies (even in the same woman) are alike. This means that although we can make tentative predictions about what women will experience in pregnancy these will only be generalisations. Where does this leave the midwife? It may appear from reading this chapter that there are no hard and fast rules in psychology. In terms of human behaviour this is unfortunately true. Psychologists may be able to make educated guesses about how people will behave in certain circumstances, but they can never be 100% accurate. Trying to make inferences about what pregnant women will think, do and feel is fraught with problems. If you try to be too prescriptive about other people's behaviour, you will inevitably run into difficulties. It is the old stereotyping problem again, although this time it is made more acceptable because it is under-pinned with research, it still does not make it right and will not necessarily help you in your everyday dealings with mothers to be.

By now you are probably thinking well, so what? What has been the point of this chapter if we cannot make generalisations? What do we actually know about pregnancy? The fact is that we do know quite a lot that can be usefully applied so long as we remember that women are unique and remain alert and sensitive to what they are **telling** us. This point is crucially important and cannot be over-emphasised. Take the research on anxiety, we know from this that some women will be anxious and need reassurance and as we saw in the study by Welles-Nystrom and de Chateau (1987), older mothers may well be more likely to experience anxiety than younger mothers. This is useful information because it draws our attention to the needs of older mothers, but we must not assume that all older mothers will be anxious, nor that younger pregnant women will not be anxious. Even with this knowledge we must still be aware of the needs of the individual and try not to make assumptions before we have given them the chance to express these needs themselves. We should not allow research to encourage us to make prejudgements about behaviour, but use the information reflectively to inform our practice and increase our sensitivity to the needs of others.

Conclusion

Pregnancy is a time of change in a woman's life and how she responds to it will depend on a range of factors. These will include whether the pregnancy is wanted, her past obstetric history, her cultural and social background and her personality. Without taking all of these factors into account it is difficult to predict beforehand how any individual will cope. As a midwife you will need to be aware of these influences and how they may interact. An understanding of the concept of locus of control and the health belief model is particularly relevant when trying to encourage pregnant women to engage in health behaviours that are likely to influence positively their own health and the health of their unborn child.

References

Bielawska-Batorowicz E (1993) The effect of previous obstetric history on women's scores on the Fetal Health Locus of Control Scale (FHLC). *J Reprod Infant Psychol* **11**: 103–6

Brindle PM, Brown MW, Brown J, Griffith HB, Turner GM (1991) Objective and subjective memory impairment in pregnancy. *Psychol Med* **21**: 647–53

Department of Health (1993) *Changing Childbirth. Report of the Expert Maternity Group.* HMSO, London

Glenn EN (1994) Social constructions of mothering: a thematic overview. In: Glenn EN, Chang G, Forcey L, eds. *Mothering: Ideolology, Experience and Ageing.* Routledge, New York

Gross H, Pattison H (1995) Cognitive failure during pregnancy. *J Reprod Infant Psychol* **13**: 17–32

Jarrahi-Zadeh A, Kane FJ, van de Castle RL, Lachenbruch PA, Ewing JA (1961) Emotional and cognitive changes in pregnancy and early puerperium. *Br J Psychiatry* **115**: 797–805

Katbamna S (2000) *Race and Chilbirth.* Oxford University Press, Buckingham

Kaplan MM (1992) *Mother's Images of Motherhood.* Routledge, New York

Kitzinger S (1989) Childbirth and society. In: Chalmers I, Enkin M, Keirse MJN, eds. *Effective Care in Pregnancy and Childbirth Vol 1.* Oxford University Press, Oxford

Labs SH, Wurtele SK (1986) Fetal health locus of control scale: Development and validation. *J Consult Clin Psychol* **54**(6): 814–19

Lever Hense A (1994) Live birth following stillbirth. In: Field PA, Marck PB, eds. *Uncertain Motherhood: Negotiating the risks of the childbearing years.* Sage, Thousand Oaks, California

Marck PB (1994) Unexpected pregnancy: the uncharted land of women's experience. In: Field PA, Marck PB, eds. *Uncertain Motherhood: Negotiating the risks of the childbearing years.* Sage, Thousand Oaks, California: 82–138

Marteau TM, Johnston M, Shaw RW, Michie S, Kidd J, New M (1988) The impact of prenatal screening and diagnostic testing upon the cognitions, emotions and behaviour of pregnant women. *J Psychosom Res* **33**(1): 7–16

Mercer RT (1995) *Becoming a Mother.* Springer, New York

Mezey GC, Bewley S (1997) Domestic violence and pregnancy. *Br Med J* **314**(5): 1295

Michelacci L, Fava GA, Grandi S, Boricelli L, Orlandi C, Trombini G (1988) Psychological reactions to ultrasound examination during pregnancy. *Psychother Psychosom* **50**(1): 1–4

Moore D (1978) The body image in pregnancy. *J Nurse Midwifery* **70**: 502–8

Norman P, Bennett P (1996) Health Locus of Control. In: Conner M, Norman P, eds. *Predicting Health Behaviour*. Open University Press, Buckingham

Oakley A (1980) *Women Confined: Towards a Sociology of Childbirth*. Martin Robertson, Oxford

Oakeley A, Hickey D, Rajan L, Rigby A (1996) Social support in pregnancy: does it have long term effects? *J Reprod Infant Psychol* **14**: 7–22

Parkes CM (1976) *Bereavement: Studies of grief in adult life*. Penguin Books, Harmondsworth

Phoenix A, Woollett A (1991) Motherhood: social construction, politics and psychology. In: Phoenix A, Woollett A, Lloyd E, eds. *Motherhood: Meanings, Practices and Ideologies*. Sage, London

Poser CM, Kassirer MR, Peyser JM (1986) Benign encephalopathy of pregnancy. *Acta Neurol Scand* **73**: 39–43

Purvin VA, Dunn DW (1987) Caffeine and the benign encephalopathy of pregnancy. *Acta Neurol Scand* **74**: 76–7

Raphael-Leff J (1991) *Psychological Processes of Childbearing*. Chapman and Hall, London

Raphael-Leff J, Perelberg RJ (eds) (1997) *Female Experience: Three generations of British women psychoanalysts on work with women*. Routledge, London

Reisch LM, Tinsley BJ (1994) Impoverished women's health locus of control and utilization of prenatal services. *J Reprod Infant Psychol* **12**: 223–32

Rhoades J (1989) Social support and the transition to the maternal role. In: Stern PN, ed. *Pregnancy and Parenting*. Hemisphere, New York: 131–41

Rossi N, Avveduti P, Rizzo N, Lorusso R (1989) Maternal stress and fetal motor behaviour: A preliminary report. *Pre- and Peri-Natal Psychol* **3**(4): 311–18

Rubin R (1961) Puerperal Change. *Nurs Outlook* **9**: 753–5

Ruggieri V, Milizia M, Romano M (1979) Effects of body image on tactile sensitivity to a tickle: A study of pregnancy. *Percept Mot Skills* **49**: 555–63

Rutter DR, Quine L, Hayward R (1988) Satisfaction with maternity care: Psychosocial factors in pregnancy outcome. *J Reprod Infant Psychol* **6**: 261–9

Sayers J (1991) *Mothering Psychoanalysis*. Hamish Hamilton, London

Schuman AN, Marteau TM (1993) Obstetricians' and midwives' contrasting perceptions of pregnancy. *J Reprod Infant Psychol* **11**: 115–18

Schuzman E (1987) Body image in pregnancy. In: Sherwen LN, ed. *Psychosocial Dimensions of the Pregnant Family*. Springer, New York: 129–56

Singh U, Saxena MSL (1991) Anxiety during pregnancy and after childbirth. *Psychol Studies* **36**(2): 108–11

Strang VR, Sullivan PL (1985) Body image attitudes during pregnancy and the postpartum period. *J Obstet Gynecol Neonatal Nurs* **14**(4): 332–7

Strickland BR (1978) Internal-external expectancies and health related behaviours. *J Consult Clin Psychol* **46**: 1192–1211

Sumner A, Waller G, Killick S, Elstein M (1993) Body image distortion in pregnancy: a pilot study of the effects of media images. *J Reprod Infant Psychol* **11**: 203–8

Tanner L (1969) Developmental tasks of pregnancy. In: Bergersen B, Andersen E, Duffer M, Lohr M, Rose H, eds. *Current Concepts in Clinical Nursing*. Mosby, St Louis, CV

Tinsley BJ, Trupin S, Owens L, Boyum LA (1993) The significance of women's pregnancy-related locus of control beliefs for adherence to recommended prenatal health regimens and pregnancy outcomes. *J Reprod Infant Psychol* **11**: 97–102

Van den Bergh BRH (1990) The influence of maternal emotions during pregnancy on fetal and neonatal behaviour. *Pre- and Peri-Natal Psychol* **5**(2): 119–30

Wallston KA, Wallston BS, DeVellis R (1978) Development of multi-dimensional health locus of control (MHLC) scales. *Health Educ Monographs* **6**: 160–70

Wallston KA (1992) Hocus-pocus, the focus isn't strictly on locus: Rotter's social learning theory modified for health. *Cognitive Ther Res* **16**: 183–99

Welles-Nystrom BL, de Chateau P (1987) Maternal age and transition to motherhood: Prenatal and perinatal assessments. *Acta Psychiatr Scand* **76**: 719–25

Winnicott DW (1958) Primary maternal preoccupation. In: Winnicott DW, ed. *Collected Papers: Through paediatrics through to psychoanalysis*. Tavistock, London: 300–5

Zimmerman-Tansella C, Bertagni P, Siani R, Micciolo R (1994) Marital relationships and somatic and psychological symptoms in pregnancy. *Soc Sci Med* **38**(4): 559–64

7

Birth: a labour of love, or baptism by fire?

As pregnant women and midwives quickly discover, women who have had babies love to tell their birth stories. Many women can give a contraction-by-contraction account of their births, even if they happened many years ago. It is rare to encounter women who have no recollection of their labour experiences. Even those who say that labour 'passed in a blur', will still try and verbally recall the details they can remember and may seek clarification of detail from their partner. Kate Jackson (1996) tells a moving story of a confused, elderly woman she met while visiting her grandmother in hospital. Jackson sat with the woman for a while and asked her if she had any children. The woman became quite lucid. She described, in detail, her one daughter who had been stillborn, and recalled the midwife who had commented that she was the most beautiful little girl that she had ever seen.

> *It was over seventy years since her baby's birth and yet those words surfaced that night through the confusion of her deteriorating mind.*

> (Jackson, 1996, p. 665)

The extent to which women recall their birth experiences has also been vividly demonstrated by Simkin (1991). She asked a small number of women what they remembered of their first birth, which had taken place between fifteen and twenty years previously. The tape-recorded interviews showed that the women had very clear recall of their birth experience and could relate what had been said by the doctors and midwives in attendance. It seems clear that labour is a very significant life event for women, whether because of positive or negative reasons, and these memories can last a lifetime.

Birth is also a time of great anxiety for many women. I always remember going to hear the obstetrician, Michel Odent talking about birth. He commented that very few studies had been done on what aspects of the environment influence women in labour, but if you looked at animals it was very clear that several things could influence labour and make it more difficult. Talking about studies on mice, he said birth complications occurred if you put them in an unfamiliar environment, moved them during labour and disturbed them by handling them. This, he pointed out, is exactly what happens to women when they are in labour. They are put in an environment which they do not know, they are often attended by people who are strangers to them and they are frequently moved around whilst in labour. A woman needs to feel relaxed in order to give birth, anxiety will inevitably prevent her from 'letting go' and behaving in a way that is most natural to her. The idea of finding ways to help a woman to feel secure during labour so that she can relax into the process of giving birth is a fundamental theme that underpins much of what is discussed in this chapter.

The emphasis throughout is on the midwife's role in supporting women through labour and birth. The stance is from the perspective of woman-centred care. This is not intended to be prescriptive: a list of what you 'should' and 'should not' do in certain situations. It is intended to enable you to be more flexible in your practice, to be aware of the importance of listening to what women are saying (both verbally and non-verbally) and to respond appropriately.

Birth as a process of transformation

Although the majority of young girls probably grow up expecting to become mothers, not all of them will achieve this aim, and those who do will probably only experience pregnancy and birth two or three times in their life. Most people will move house more often than they give birth. Birth may be natural, but it is still an uncommon experience for each woman.

Despite this, birth is a process of transformation. For a woman giving birth to her first child, the transformation is to that of 'mother', but even if she has children already, she is still changed by the addition of a new child to her family. Raphael-Leff (1991) discusses the transition from daughterhood to motherhood, and states that women need, 'warm cherishing acceptance' (p. 281) to enable them to make this transition. The midwife who supports a woman in labour can provide this acceptance. In a later text Raphael-Leff (1993) describes birth as an uncoupling, in which the pregnant woman has to relinquish the imaginary baby for a real baby. The midwife who has an understanding of some of the psychological implications of the birth process will give women the opportunity to acknowledge their feelings, some of which might be ambivalent, while providing reassurance that these are normal.

One author has suggested that:

> *There is a tension between the views of birth as a life crisis and pregnancy as a natural physiological and psychological process.*

(Moore, 1997, p. 51)

I am not sure that birth should be viewed as a life crisis but it is certainly true that the birth of a child marks a great change in a woman's life. The psychological changes that women undergo in the process cannot be underestimated. As we saw in *Chapter 6*, the process of transformation begins in pregnancy, and is consolidated by birth. This process continues throughout the postnatal period and beyond.

A small piece of qualitative research demonstrated that women experience birth as a unique event: several described a changing sense of self on becoming a mother. The authors also liken birth to a journey and comment that:

> *What you take on a journey influences how you perceive it.*

(Halldorsdottir and Karlsdottir, 1996, p. 57)

In other words, women's cultural background and personal beliefs, as well as their life experiences will inform and influence their birth experience. For example, Sheiner *et al* (1999) found in their study of Jewish and Bedouin women, differences in pain perception during and after labour. Midwives cannot change these beliefs (nor should they try to) but in attempting to understand them more fully they can support the woman more ably. The difference and unique beliefs surrounding birth are not discussed here, but further reading is recommended, particularly the work of Schott and Henley (1996) and Katbamna (2000).

Issues of pain and anxiety

In general, women expect labour to be painful. As one author graphically explains:

The most obvious and compelling feature of labour is the physical pain caused by moving a three kilogram baby out of the body through a fairly small opening using only muscular contractions as the propelling force.

(Kirkman, 1998, p. 328)

This pain has a physiological origin resulting from the stimulation and response of sensory receptors but there is a psychological component to the pain as well. The physiological aspect of pain is described briefly below. For more detailed texts on the topic see Mander, 1998; Moore, 1997; Yerby, 2000.

Physiological labour pain is caused by contraction of the uterine muscles, dilatation of the cervix, distension and stretching of the lower segment of the uterus, and traction and pressure on the pelvic organs and nerves. These all cause the transmission of noxious (ie. possibly pain producing) stimuli to the central nervous system warning of actual or potential tissue damage (Lowe, 1996). This rudimentary description of the transmission of labour pain does not take into account the subjective experience of pain by the individual. The gate control theory described by Melzack and Wall (1965) attempted to explain the individual's perception of pain. As Melzack and Wall (1988) elaborated in a later text, levels of pain do not always reflect the extent of tissue damage or injury: minor injuries may cause severe pain and vice versa. Moreover, pain cannot be described as a single sensation but has many dimensions. The gate control theory suggests that pain can only travel to the brain when the 'gate' within the grey matter of the dorsal horn of the spinal cord is open. The purpose of pain relief is to close this 'gate' (Moore, 1994). The gate may be closed not only by pharmacological means, but also by other strategies, such as massage and transcutaneous nerve stimulation (TENS) which release the body's own endorphins.

The perception of pain, whatever its source, may be affected by psychological as well as physical factors (Melzack and Wall, 1965). Perceptions of pain have been classified into three groups, indicating both physiological and psychological elements (Moore, 1997). The sensory qualities of pain are those that describe the physical perception of the pain, such as cramping, stabbing or sharp. The affective qualities describe the effect of the pain on emotions and motivation, such as exhausting or frightening. The evaluative qualities of the pain are the words used to describe the whole experience, such as intense or unbearable. It is the affective element of pain that may most easily be alleviated by psychological support in labour.

Attitudes to pain can also be influential in the experience of labour and these can be affected by a woman's cultural background. In many modernised Western cultures, including Britain, we tend to see the pain of childbirth as abnormal, something that needs to be controlled and alleviated. As doctors and midwives have the control of pain-relieving medication perhaps it is also the case that women have to demonstrate that they are in pain before they are actually given pain relief (Squire, 2000). Cultural attitudes to pain vary. This is not to suggest that other cultures do not feel pain, rather that the experience of pain is interpreted in a different light (Crafter, 2000). This difference in attitude may strongly influence the entire birth experience.

The concept of the emotional pain of labour has been used to describe the emotional or psychological factors that may affect the birth experience (Kirkman, 1998; Moore, 1997). Moore points out that the role of the midwife is not solely to try and alleviate physical pain (with its physiological cause) either by pharmacological or other means, but also to consider other aspects of pain relief. She highlights the fact that a woman's perception of pain is influenced by psychological factors. Similarly, it has been shown that anxiety is associated with increased pain (Lowe, 1996). How can the midwife use her knowledge of these factors to alleviate someone's pain?

Niven (1994) found a positive correlation between attendance at childbirth preparation classes and lower levels of pain. There are alternative explanations for this finding. One possibility is that women who attend classes are inherently different from those who do not and have a higher 'pain threshold'. Another explanation could be due to the fact that women learn coping strategies in antenatal classes that enable them to deal with the pain. This explanation is borne out by a more recent study by McCrea *et al* (2000). These researchers administered a questionnaire to 100 women and found that antenatal training predicted feelings of personal control in pain relief. Niven's research demonstrated that women who learned breathing exercises experienced reduced levels of affective pain as well as the overall pain of birth. (Affective pain, as discussed earlier, is the effect of pain on emotions and motivation.) Niven goes on to describe other coping strategies that women might be taught, such as distraction, eg. counting backwards from 100; imagery (concentrating on a vivid image, such as a beautiful beach); or thinking positively about the pain (what Niven describes as 'reversing the affect' of pain). Her research indicates that women who use distraction or who think positively, report significantly lower levels of labour pain. Similarly,

Green *et al* (1998) found that women who used breathing exercises throughout labour found these very useful and were more likely to be satisfied with their birth experience.

It is important to bear in mind that not all women seek total relief from the physical pain of labour. Capogna *et al* (1996) found that maternal satisfaction was highest when effective epidural analgesia was provided and conclude that this significantly improves the experience of childbirth. A sample of the questionnaire is not supplied, so it is not possible to know how questions were framed. These may have only asked about satisfaction with pain relief; women may expect more from the birth experience than the provision of adequate analgesia. One author has noted that for some women:

> *The labour and birth process is viewed as a developmental event... the mastery of which leads to an increase of self-esteem and personal strength.*
>
> (Lowe, 1996, p. 83)

Some women will simply want strategies to enable them to cope with the pain. Lowe goes on to comment that 'management' of labour pain suggests an element of control.

> *The provider must realise that labour pain belongs to the woman experiencing it, and management of the pain also belongs to her. What the provider can and must do is engage in a cooperative effort with the woman to provide whatever external tools she requires to manage her experience of pain.*
>
> (Lowe, 1996, p. 87)

I would go one step further and suggest that skilled midwifery care can enable women to use their own *internal* strategies to cope with pain. As Niven (1994) has noted, coping strategies, such as relaxation training, breathing techniques and distraction all help to alleviate and lessen pain, but another important factor is the development and maintenance of a good relationship between the midwife and the woman which allows her to utilise her own coping skills.

It is important to remember that each woman is an individual and needs the opportunity to explain what she is feeling. It is impossible for the midwife to judge how bad she thinks the woman's pain is. As we have already seen, the experience of pain is subjective and is influenced by both internal and external factors. Labour pain is as bad as an individual woman perceives it to be and there are significant individual differences in pain perception. Similarly, the midwife should not put pressure on a woman to have analgesia because she perceives the contractions to be strong and painful or because she does not think the woman is coping. As the pain cannot be felt by the midwife it is impossible for her to infer what the woman in labour is feeling. Hunt and Symonds (1995) explain how midwives use the term 'nigglers' to describe women who are not perceived to be in 'proper' labour, yet these women may be experiencing extreme discomfort and their pain needs to be acknowledged. Conversely, it cannot be assumed that because a woman is quiet or compliant that she is not in pain or distress.

It has been suggested that some health professionals see pain as a symptom 'to be managed, regulated, restrained' (Raphael-Leff, 1991). While no one would want to see a labouring woman in pain and do nothing to help, the proficiency lies in offering appropriate, sensitive help. The skilled midwife will recognise and respond to each woman's needs, understanding that those needs may change as labour progresses. Such a flexible approach might enable the woman to deal with her pain in the way that she feels to be most appropriate. This could be through pharmacological analgesia but it may simply mean suggesting going for a walk, or offering some other distraction.

Moore (1997) has discussed the cognitive appraisal that each individual makes of a painful event, cognition being the understanding that we have of pain. A woman's life experiences and her feelings about giving birth will affect her cognition of labour pain. In addition, the people who support a woman in labour, whether her friends and family or the midwife, will all interpret the woman's pain differently. We need to be careful not to let our cognitive processes get in the way of the understanding of the individual. Moore (1997) comments:

> *Behaviour associated with pain in labour is often considered unacceptable by those surrounding the labouring woman because they find her vocalisation uncomfortable, disquieting and even embarrassing; this can lead to a belief that it should be reduced as soon as possible... Pain relief is therefore sometimes encouraged not to reduce the woman's pain, but merely to comfort those who are observing.*

(p. 49)

Anecdotal experience suggests that the lack of soundproofing in most hospitals may also influence the use of analgesia. Pain relief is sometimes offered on a busy labour ward to ease the discomfort of those who might be listening outside. Remarks have been overheard about the noises women make in labour and disparaging comments about the midwife in attendance for not 'keeping the woman quiet'. Raphael-Leff (1993) also comments that midwives often strive to keep women quiet.

Of course women should not be screaming out in fear and agony but there is certainly a place for noise in labour. It can be helpful and constructive and enable a woman to feel more in control. Green *et al* (1998) found that women did not equate making a lot of noise with losing control, and did not feel less fulfilled if they did make a lot of noise. Women should not be discouraged from making a noise just to relieve the distress of others. After all, vocalising might actually help her to cope with the strange sensations she is experiencing. Green *et al* did discover that women who felt they made a lot of noise were less satisfied with their birth experience. I wonder whether this was because of their own discomfiture or because of perceived disapproval or embarrassment on the part of the midwives, or other birth attendants? However, the authors do not explore this finding in detail.

One woman, writing about her own experience of the hospital birth in water of her first child, attended by an independent midwife, writes vividly about the beneficial effects she felt from making a noise in labour:

> *As well as the water, which I found wonderfully relaxing between contractions, I used Rescue Remedy to cope with the pain, and also making a lot of noise! I have a loud, trained voice, as I am a singer and I enjoyed making all the strange noises I made to express the pain.*

(Budden, 1998, p. 16)

The relief of pain in labour is an important part of the midwife's role but this should be directed at assessing and responding to each woman's unique needs. The terms fetal distress and maternal distress are commonly heard on the labour ward, but we need to be careful that we do not offer women pain relief because of 'midwife distress'. The provision of sensitive, supportive care throughout labour undoubtedly has analgesic properties that may be just as powerful as any pharmacological preparation.

It has been suggested that one of the most important psychological factors to influence a woman's perception of pain is her sense of control (Moore, 1997; McCrea *et al*, 2000) and this may have a profound influence on her birth experience.

The importance of control in labour

The report of the Expert Maternity Group (DoH, 1993) stated that choice, continuity and control should be available to all women using the maternity services. These three 'Cs' have been much discussed over the past few years: new styles of care have been developed in order to try and achieve greater continuity, and the concept of client choice is now widely acknowledged (Hundley *et al*, 1997). Both continuity and choice will be referred to throughout this chapter but the focus here is on the subject of control. In *Chapter 6* we considered the concept of locus of control and the significance that this has for health. Green *et al* (1998) in a large study investigating women's experiences of childbirth, conclude that feelings of control, particularly feeling *in* control of what staff are doing, are of particular significance to women. Their research demonstrated that although other factors, such as the length of labour or perceptions of pain are important at different times during the birth, issues of control seem to be consistently important.

As we have already seen in the chapter on social influence, all human behaviour is subject to control, whether self-control or control exerted by an outside force. During labour, when women may find themselves in pain in unfamiliar surroundings, when they are also experiencing a high level of anxiety, it is very easy to feel out of control. This is likely to be exacerbated if the labouring woman thinks that other people are making important decisions about the management of her labour without discussion and consultation.

Women's perceptions of control during labour

Everyone wants to believe that they are able to influence what happens to them. When people feel powerless about their lives, they are likely to become worried, anxious and depressed. In general, we feel that we have control, however, in a hospital situation it is easy to feel that you have no control because you are in an unfamiliar and often frightening situation, where the professionals hold the balance of power.

Although you might not want to acknowledge it, midwives hold much more control than they think. Consider for a moment the subtle interactions between client and professional that are used to retain balance of control. Even relatively simple decisions can have a powerful influence over a woman in labour. For example, when you are admitting someone on the labour ward you might allocate Jane X to room 4, even though rooms 5 and 8 are empty. You are in control of the room she will be in to have her baby. You ask Jane what has been happening and then you say, 'OK, I'd just like to feel how the baby is lying, can you just get up on the bed'. Jane might prefer to stay upright but it is hard for her as the 'visitor' to state her wishes, so you remain in control (remember what we said about authority?). These may seem rather trivial examples, but they illustrate the kind of control that practitioners have over women. Midwives are usually aware of the extent to which they are controlled and dominated, both by the medical profession and their employers. It is not always so easy to recognise the control that midwives can have over women in their care.

The ways in which women define feelings of being in control varies from one individual to another. Niven (1994) drawing conclusions from her own research studying the coping strategies of fifty-one labouring women noted striking differences. She found that some women defined 'control' in terms of control over the management of the labour, such as being involved in the decision-making processes, while others were concerned with feeling 'out of control' and 'showing themselves up'. Another group of women was concerned with control over the birth process such as the length of labour. Raphael-Leff (1993) suggests that in order to retain feelings of being in control some women want an active birth, while others opt for predictability and choose a 'high-tech' birth. Control means different things to different people. In a small-scale qualitative study involving fifteen women, Weaver (1998) found that the subjects in her research wanted to achieve a balance, taking control where they wished, but relinquishing control where they felt this to be appropriate.

It seems both obvious and reasonable that women should want to be involved in decisions about the extent to which they take control. It also seems reasonable that women will, at times, look to the professionals, whether the midwife or obstetrician to take control. Handing control back to the midwife can be the most important way in which a woman exerts control, if it is her own choice. However, as Weaver noted in her study, women may sometimes be given control without choice. Giving a woman more control than she wants may be just as detrimental to her sense of well being as the maintenance of complete control by the health professionals. As Niven (1992) points out, personal control and professional control do not have to be antagonistic concepts and can be both mutually supportive and beneficial. But, there is ample evidence that this balance is often not achieved. Perhaps one of the most essential skills of midwifery practice is knowing when to take control and when to hand this back again. This can only be achieved through excellent communication, listening to what women are saying, being sensitive to their behaviour and responding to both verbal and non-verbal cues.

One way in which women may be encouraged to express their wishes or preferences is in the writing of birth plans. Green *et al* (1998) found that the women in their study expressed a wish for good communication and a flexible approach from staff, some women felt that birth plans would obstruct this whereas others felt that they were helpful. Less than half of the women questioned who had written a birth plan had found this beneficial. Was this perhaps because of the way in which the plans were presented? As Price (1998) points out, the use of a preset format, with a list of questions to answer, may restrict, rather than enhance women's choice. She goes on to comment that systems of care that allow women to be cared for by someone they know may eliminate the need for birth plans. This does not mean, that women should not be encouraged to write down their wishes. Some women will find it helpful to write things down and will find that this enables them to clarify their thoughts in their own mind. As one author has stated:

> *It takes very little insight to see that birth plans are an expression of anxiety, fear, hopes and expectations. We cannot divorce the woman from these aspirations and feelings by implying that she should not write them down, because they will still be there, whether or not they are written or read.*

> (Rogers, 1998, p. 524)

Weaver (1998) notes that not all women feel comfortable with the idea of a **written** birth plan. The purpose of birth plans is not to create yet another procedure with which women must comply. They should be flexible and optional, offered to all women with the understanding that not everyone will choose to use them. Birth plans are just one of the many tools that can be used as an aid to discussion, rather than as a substitute for good communication. Like all tools they need to be used sensitively and appropriately.

Weaver also points out that knowledge and information will affect **perceptions** of power and women may see midwives as both informed and knowledgeable. Some women may feel reassured by this and will feel that they can trust the people who are caring for them in labour. Bluff and Holloway (1994) undertook a small piece of qualitative research examining women's birth experiences. Their data demonstrated that women trust midwives because the latter are seen as experts who 'know best'. This belief would seem to indicate that women who trust their midwives may be happy for decisions to be made for them by these 'experts'. However, Bluff and Holloway go on to point out that women want to be actively involved in decision making, and to retain a sense of control, even when they trust the staff completely. Green *et al* (1998) undertook a large, prospective study of women's experiences of childbirth. The results of their work demonstrated that:

> *Positive psychological outcomes were associated with the belief that the right thing had happened rather than with the activity itself.*

(p. 249)

For example, a woman might have written on her birth plan that she wanted no pain relief but ended up with an epidural, but was happy because she felt supported and informed in making her decision. Another woman in the same situation might have been very unhappy because she felt that she was browbeaten into accepting the epidural. This highlights for me the awesome amount of power that midwives hold. It is a huge responsibility to ensure that this power is used wisely and that positions of trust are not abused.

Environmental influences and the perception of control

The hospital environment

Institutions, such as hospitals, have been noted to be centres of power and control (Illich, 1976) and may develop mechanisms to defend and protect their practices. The use of hospital policies and protocols should, if based on sound evidence, serve to protect both users and employees of the maternity services. All too often these policies may be used to continue practices that are based on no evidence at all. One very obvious example is the widespread use of the admissions trace, that is, a cardiotocograph (CTG) done on admission to record the baby's heartbeat for a given length of time. There is no evidence that continuous monitoring improves the outcome for babies and yet this is common practice on many labour wards. Such practices send out clear messages to women that when they enter the hospital they are no longer in control and, moreover, that they can no longer be trusted to look after the baby themselves — they need the hospital staff to do this for them.

The environment in which women give birth may affect the balance of power. One writer, noted that:

> *Women are the strangers or 'guests', the professionals are the hosts within the hospital.*

> (Sherr, 1995, p. 187)

The machinery and equipment used in the hospital serve to stress this relationship even more strongly as does the uniform worn by midwives. In contrast, women are usually expected to wear night-clothes and lie passively on the bed, further emphasising their complete absence of power. Price (1988) notes that psychologically, as well as physically, lying down in labour might have serious drawbacks: women may feel more ' themselves' if upright, walking or sitting. Lying in bed, particularly in a hospital, may be associated with illness and the woman in labour may accept the 'sick' role. She may feel less assertive, more childlike and more willing to accept decisions made on her behalf. The unfamiliar noises, smells and faces that surround a woman in labour may create further dis-orientation and a subsequent loss of control. The solution to such difficulties is not always easy although hospitals and midwives are constantly trying to make the labour room more 'normal' and home-like. But, as Sherr (1995) points out, attempts to change some of these factors may be mere tokenism. Moving from uniform to 'mufti' may help some women but may actually disorientate others who, surrounded by a sea of unfamiliar faces, do not know who to turn to for advice. Similarly, knocking at the door of a labour room is polite but how often is entry denied? Garcia and Garforth (1990) commenting on the level of power and control held by health professionals on a labour ward state:

> *If someone did knock, it would seem strange for a parent*
> *to answer because the room is not 'theirs'.*

(p. 176)

Most women enter labour with some apprehension (Price, 1988). Labour is always a strange and unpredictable event, even for the woman who has children already. The environment in which women give birth may exacerbate this sense of apprehension. Most women are only occasional 'visitors' to the hospital and labour ward and will suffer a sense of disorientation and alienation within this unfamiliar setting. One particular facet of care in labour, pointed out by Kirkham (1989) is that women in labour are usually cared for in single rooms which means that they cannot get any orientation from other women. Subsequently, they are particularly dependent on staff. In her study of midwives and information giving during labour, Kirkham notes that women want information with which to orientate themselves as to time, place and likely events and describe their ideal midwife as someone who provides this information. Women who receive this information will feel more confident and in control. In contrast, women who feel disorientated may feel less in control and more fearful about the whole process.

> *Labour is often experienced by a woman as an inner loss*
> *of control over her own body and [is] therefore*
> *intrinsically distressing, with or without associated pain.*
> *If the woman also feels she has no control over her*
> *immediate environment and no idea what is going to*
> *happen next the fear associated with the loss of control*
> *becomes even greater.*

(Price, 1988, p. 40)

Home births: the advantages of a familiar environment

Women who give birth in hospital have less control over some of their actions. Being in an alien environment they may feel they have to 'ask permission' before they can go to the toilet, get a drink or go for a walk. The balance of power is very different at home as the woman is on her own territory: in this instance it is the midwives who have to familiarise themselves with a different environment. Garcia and Garforth (1990) comment that the difference at home is that, while parents may seek advice and encouragement from midwives, they probably will not seek permission.

Weaver (1998) suggests that the environment in which women give birth also has a powerful effect and may influence perceptions of control. A typical hospital labour room tends to be full of machines such as the CTG monitor and the resuscitaire, with the bed dominating the room. It may be hard for a woman to be active and upright in labour unless this option is offered to her. This does not mean, of course, that women who give birth at home automatically feel as though they are in control, or that women in hospital feel a lesser sense of control. I only use this as an example of the profound effect that the environment may have in exerting control over a woman's behaviour.

Women in Britain have less choice over the place of birth than they used to, with the closure of small units and maternity homes (Pollard and Robotham, 1998). New initiatives, such as the implementation of midwifery group practices and midwife-led care, and the development of birth centres within and outside the NHS should increase the options open to women. Control over the place of birth should be every woman's right.

Control and satisfaction

An understanding of some of the issues involved in the giving or withholding of control is of fundamental importance as research has demonstrated that women's satisfaction with their birth experience is closely linked with feelings of control. Simkin (1991) demonstrated that feelings of control were strongly related to long-term satisfaction and feelings of self-worth. In contrast, Green *et al* (1998) found that women who felt out of control, were less likely to find the birth a fulfilling experience. Halldorsdottir and Karlsdottir (1996) undertook a phenomenological study of fourteen women's experience of birth. The women interviewed expressed a need for caring and understanding in labour, and also a wish for control of themselves and the birth process. The interviewees described the impact of the midwife on the birth experience and stated that a midwife can turn a difficult birth into a positive experience or vice versa. A lack of caring, support and communication may lead women to experience a sense of loss of control. Conversely, good support may enable a woman to perceive the birth, whatever the outcome as a positive life experience.

Importance of control — a summary

What can be gleaned from this understanding of the importance of control in labour? As Weaver (1998) points out, women's desire for control is complex; not all women will want the same degree of control in childbirth. Women's perceptions and wishes for control may change and fluctuate throughout the labour. Good midwifery care will recognise that each woman is unique, each woman perceives and defines control differently, and each woman will want a different measure of control.

Halldorsdottir and Karlsdottir (1996) found that some women viewed birth as a journey. This view can be turned into a useful analogy to describe the role of the midwife in maintaining the balance of control during labour. Critics (art critics, theatre critics and the like) sometimes defend their role by saying that, 'although they do not know how to drive the car, they know how to navigate'. A film critic may never have made a film in her life, but she understands the process and feels that she can point out the flaws when the process is incorrect. A midwife is not there to point out the flaws in the birth process but, understanding the physiology and psychology of birth, she can help a woman to 'navigate' through the experience. Whatever intervention might be necessary, it is the woman herself who gives birth and she can be seen as the 'driver' along the journey. The midwife should see herself as a very useful, map-reading passenger. On a good journey she may be able to sit back, and leave the driver to it, while remaining alert to any unanticipated hazards along the way. If the 'driver' becomes tired she can offer moral support and, although she cannot take over the journey, she can see herself as a driving instructor who has access to dual-controls. She can give guidance when she sees that the road ahead may be rough and, because she has the skills, she can deal with unexpected problems, much as a good passenger in a car knows how to change a wheel. Control over the birth is subject to ongoing discussion, but it is the woman who should be in charge of this negotiation.

Birth companions and the birth environment

The hospital is an unfamiliar environment to most women in labour and being admitted to hospital may carry with it a sense of profound anxiety. In the midst of all of these new experiences, a woman may search for the familiar with which she can orientate herself. Most familiar of all are the chosen birth companions who support her in labour. She may also seek help and reassurance from the midwives. Both these groups, the 'lay' and the professional, can provide invaluable support that will enable a woman to have the birth experience that she wants.

What about birth companions? What is the effect of their presence at the birth? To have a chosen companion who she can trust and who knows, from previous discussion, exactly what she wants must be an immense source of comfort to women in labour. Niven (1992) found in her research study that women who positively welcomed the presence of their partner at the birth also had lower levels of labour pain when compared with other women. The partner also needs some support from the midwife since, for them, labour and birth are just as much an 'unknown' experience as for the woman herself. The partner, whether male or female, is emotionally involved and likely to be very concerned about the woman and her baby. They will have to deal with their own anxieties and uncertainties and any feelings of disorientation in an unfamiliar environment. In addition, concern about whether they will cope, distress at seeing their partner in pain and possibly behaving in an atypical fashion, and their feelings towards the baby, which may be ambivalent will be influential. They may feel inhibited about showing intimacy with their partner in the presence of a 'professional' and may, as a result, not offer the physical tactile support that their partner wants. The role of the partner and other supporters may be crucial to the woman's birth experience: the midwife is there to enable them to fulfil that role.

Although it is now common practice for the father of the baby to attend the birth, there are still some couples who would prefer this not to happen. Niven (1992) found that 16% of the women interviewed did not find the presence of their male partner helpful. Michel Odent has written that the presence of the male partner may be disruptive to the birth process, and argues that birth is traditionally an all-female event. Although not everyone would agree with this position, his claim does raise the question of whether social pressure now demands that all fathers should attend the birth, whatever the personal feelings of the man himself. Similarly, it may be difficult for the woman to verbalise her wishes if she would prefer another birth companion. Midwives need to be sensitive to each relationship and allow each family unit to decide for themselves what is best, giving 'permission' for individuals to leave the room if this seems appropriate.

It would be wrong to assume that all women have a male partner. It would be equally wrong to try and 'second guess' the relationship between the woman and her chosen birth companion(s). A male companion may not be the woman's partner or the father of the baby, whereas a female companion may be her mother, sister, lesbian lover or friend. It requires sensitivity on the part of the midwife to make the partner feel welcome, giving the couple the opportunity to disclose their relationship if they choose.

Role of midwives

A study in Dublin (O'Driscoll and Meagher, 1980) demonstrated that women who have constant support and encouragement from a midwife or, more usually a student midwife, require minimal analgesia, even when their labour is being actively managed and augmented. Such support is rarely achieved on many labour wards in Britain where midwives may be required to care for two or even three labouring women simultaneously. Investigations into alternative systems of care, such as 'one-to-one' midwifery, case-load midwifery and team midwifery have all sought to overcome some of the more frequent problems that women face, in particular, fragmented care and lack of a known carer in labour. Evaluations of these systems by the women have, in general, been favourable, and have had some impact on 'measurable outcomes' that phrase beloved by auditors. The system of 'one-to-one' care that was established in London for example, demonstrated that women receiving such care were significantly less likely to use epidural anaesthesia during labour (Page *et al*, 1996). A review of the literature carried out by Waldenstrom and Turnbull (1998) looked at the data from seven randomised trials. The trials identified looked at 9148 women in all. The authors considered the number of interventions in women who received continuity of midwifery care compared to those who received 'standard' maternity care. They found that continuity of midwifery care was associated with less use of obstetric interventions during labour such as induction, augmentation of labour, electronic fetal monitoring, instrumental vaginal delivery and episiotomy.

The work of Green *et al* (1998) demonstrated that women were significantly more satisfied with the birth experience when they had one midwife who was with them throughout labour. This satisfaction was not related to having met the midwife antenatally. Similarly,

Garcia *et al* (1998) found in their research that a large proportion of women questioned (48%) stated that it was very important to have the same staff with them throughout the labour and birth. In contrast, only 24% said it was important to have met the staff before the birth. These findings may well relate to women's prior expectations. That is, if women have not been led to believe that they will meet a known midwife at the birth they will not be disappointed when this does not happen. As Garcia *et al* go on to point out, continuity of carer is usually related to expectations, ie. if women have been led to believe that they will have the same carer throughout their pregnancy and intrapartum this becomes very important to them. As a result, if their expectations are not met, they may be disappointed. The research by Green *et al* and Garcia *et al* suggests that it is important to women's birth experience to have a feeling of constancy around the time of birth — a period of intense physical and emotional experiences. Perhaps employers need to address the question of providing more constant care throughout labour.

Continuity of care

These discussions explore what women may find helpful in the way of midwifery support in labour, but what are the psychological mechanisms that underlie this need for good support? Most people have an inherent need for security and are more likely to feel safe in familiar surroundings with familiar people. On a day-to-day basis we all have many signposts that provide this security and reassurance. These include the familiar landscape of our homes and all the many activities that mark out the course of a typical day. The hourly news bulletins on the radio, for example, is just one of hundreds of events that may give a sense of pattern and predictability to the average commuter driving to work. Women in labour often feel very vulnerable. They may be in considerable pain, and worried about their baby and their ability to cope. If all the familiar signposts of their everyday lives are removed their vulnerability increases. If a woman can be helped to feel safe she will undoubtedly have a better birth experience.

With the increasing pressure on midwives in hospital, questions have been raised about the most appropriate support for women. Research has indicated that women will feel more secure if they have a constant companion who stays with them throughout labour. This could, of course, be the midwife, but it does not have to be. Meta-analysis of eleven randomised controlled trials suggested that the presence of a doula (a trained layperson) who provides continuous support to a woman in labour may improve both obstetric and neonatal outcomes (Klaus and Kennell, 1997). An earlier study by Kennell *et al* (1991) also suggested that women supported by a doula required less intervention in labour and used less analgesia. However Hodnett (2000) looked at fourteen randomised trials which considered the effects of continuous support during labour provided by either healthcare workers or lay people. In all, 5000 women were involved in the trials. The findings indicated that the continuous presence of a support person reduced the likelihood of medication for pain relief, operative vaginal delivery, Caesarean section and a five-minute Apgar score of less than seven. Six of the trials also evaluated the mother's view of childbirth experience and results favoured the group who had received continuous support.

These studies indicate that continuous support during labour has a profound impact on a woman's birth experience, but how can midwives ensure that women have this support? Is it feasible for midwives to provide this; or do we need to acknowledge that in some situations this is best provided by someone else? It is, after all, much cheaper to provide a doula who has little formal training, particularly if she then has an impact on the length of labour and amount of analgesia used.

The report of the Expert Maternity Group (DoH, 1993) states that the midwife should provide low key support to a woman and her family when a birth is going well, giving more sophisticated care if complications occur.This emphasis on low key is absolutely crucial. A small phenomenological study by Berg *et al* (1996) demonstrated that women expressed a wish for support and encouragement from the midwife, but wanted this to be on their own terms. They wanted the midwife to recognise them as an individual, and to provide constant ongoing support that did not become an attempt by the midwife to dominate the whole event. Birth does not belong to the midwife — it is the woman's birth and we are privileged to attend. One independent practitioner has put this succinctly. She has stated that she really feels that she has done a good job if, when she leaves the house after a birth, the couple hardly notice her going because they are so wrapped up in their new baby (Coyle, 2000). I have heard the concept of 'masterly inactivity' used to describe the competent and confident midwife. This is the practitioner who is prepared to 'sit on her hands' giving the woman support and encouragement, while also believing in the woman's own ability to give birth herself. I am not saying that the midwife should do nothing, but a birth where we sit back and watch and wait demands just as much skill as a very complex birth. There is a place for intervention but this should be appropriate and sensitive not a taking over of the whole process.

The physical environment

The impact of the physical environment on the experience of childbirth also needs to be considered. The safety of home birth for women with no complications cannot be disputed (Olsen, 1997). From a psychological point of view it seems logical that women will labour most effectively in an environment in which they feel safe. As I pointed out earlier in this chapter, pain is a complex sensory experience that has psychological as well as physical origins. Women who feel secure in their environment and with their birth companions may produce more endorphins and so cope more effectively with the pain of labour. Raphael-Leff (1991) suggests that women at home are less likely to feel inhibited because they are in a familiar environment and so feel more in control.

As Weaver (1998) has pointed out, midwives need to be reflexive practitioners. That is, they must take into account their own position as an 'actor' or participant in the woman's birth. The midwife should be aware of her own feelings about the people she is with. Undoubtedly these feelings will change with each birth: the dynamics created with a couple-partnership will always be unique on that occasion. What are the midwife's own life experiences, moral codes, beliefs etc that may affect her behaviour? What sort of day has she had/is she having? Has she had a row with her partner or has she just come from a wonderful session of lovemaking? What are her day-to-day concerns and anxieties? What does she feel about the colleagues she is with — does she get on with the midwife in charge, or does she find her domineering? Does she feel supported at work or does she feel that she is working in isolation? All these factors and more will affect the way midwives behave on a day-to-day and hour-to-hour basis. The points raised above are used just as a reminder that the experience of birth can be affected by the relationships between all the participants, including the mother, her companions, and the midwife. These relationships can be understood by the communication between all the individuals concerned.

Communication during labour

The subject of communication has been discussed in depth in *Chapter 5*. It is, however, worth considering some of the particular issues that may have an impact on communication during labour and birth. Women's experiences of labour can be greatly enhanced by psychological support from midwives, and their satisfaction with the birth experience will depend on interactions with the staff (Taylor and Copstick, 1985). One way in which midwives provide psychological support is by listening to women, and talking to them in a language they understand. The fundamental importance of good communication in labour cannot be overstated.

The work of Kirkham in the 1980s is often quoted when discussing issues of communication in labour. Kirkham's observational study of over 100 births demonstrated the ways in which language was variously used to coerce, judge or reassure women. As Kirkham points out, words of reassurance such as the phrase 'don't worry' often more closely resemble a denial of a woman's apprehensions. She also noted the extent to which midwives use 'verbal asepsis' first described by Kitzinger (1978) to block information and conversations. A later ethnographic study by Hunt noted a similar phenomenon:

Woman: *My back really aches, is that normal?*
Midwife: *Yes.*
Woman: *What did that doctor mean when he said, 'She'll probably need some help'?*
Midwife: *Don't worry about that.*

(Hunt and Symonds, 1994, p. 108)

This brief exchange demonstrates the extent to which midwives may control the information that they give to women, avoiding questions and providing scant reassurance. Weaver (1998) also discussed the problems created when midwives block information to women. She points out that this is not the only communication problem, however, and that midwives sometimes use coercive language to gain consent from women prior to a procedure. A typical example of coercion is the use of the rhetorical question, where the midwife may think she is giving the woman an option ('I'll just pop you on the monitor, OK?') but where the woman has little alternative but to agree.

The challenge for midwives is to make communication really effective with each individual, bearing in mind the points made earlier about the power relationships that exist between staff and women. The consequences of this power relationship and the fact that most women give birth in an alien environment attended by unfamiliar people, undoubtedly impacts on issues of communication.

The use of medical jargon

One barrier to effective communication may be the language used by midwives and other health carers. The use of medical terminology and abbreviations will almost certainly heighten the sense of alienation that the women might experience in labour. Consider some of the common phrases that may be overheard on a typical labour ward:

> *It's cephalic* (This, I have to confess is my particular bug bear. I don't consider myself a Latin scholar. What on earth is wrong with saying the baby is coming head first?)
> *She's been fully for an hour, but there's no sign of descent.*
> *I've done an ARM and I'm going to put up synto.*

While none of these phrases may be addressed to the woman herself, they are often used within her hearing. What on earth is she to make of them? One vivid, though anecdotal example of this occurred in one of my student's midwifery training. A woman had overheard the expression, 'The baby's a bit flat' and asked if this meant that the baby would be very thin.

Women who attend antenatal classes may learn some of the 'lingo' of birth, and may find it relatively easy to express themselves. Some women are very articulate and assertive whether or not they have been to classes. But as we have seen, even the most assertive woman may be intimidated and therefore silenced by the alien hospital environment. As Weaver (1998) points out, women who gain knowledge about birth from informal sources, such as family and friends, may not have the language to express their wishes. It should not be the responsibility of the woman, however, to have to learn a coded language or niceties of behaviour that 'earn' her the right to information.

The use of unfamiliar words and phrases can act as an exclusionary strategy (Macdonald, 1995) to create a barrier between the 'professionals' and the women. Sometimes this is done with the best of intentions. The midwife may not inform a woman of complications that are occurring during labour as she may wish to prevent unnecessary anxiety. Kirkham's study (1989) demonstrated that women wish to be informed if things seem to be 'going wrong'. Similarly, a study carried out in Sweden studying women's experiences of complicated childbirth demonstrated that women wished to be given information even when this was unpleasant (Berg and Dahlberg, 1998).

Having said this, we cannot assume that all women want to be given the same level of information. I do not want to suggest that midwives would patronise women by trying to 'guess' what level of information they might want to be given but there is a need to be sensitive to each woman's wishes. The important thing to remember is not to act as a barrier to information, but to create an environment where women feel they can ask questions if they want and know they will be answered with honesty and respect. Women who require intervention in labour need to understand the reason for, and appropriateness of, that intervention. This can only be achieved with good communication. Green *et al* (1998) found that when women had things 'done to them' with inadequate discussion, they were dissatisfied with their care, whereas when an agreement was reached after full discussion the women were much more satisfied. Good communication requires that information is shared fully and honestly without resorting to economy with the truth. A midwife may, for example, offer to rupture a woman's membranes during labour, stating that this will 'speed things up'. This may sound attractive to the woman but the midwife is being economical with the truth if she does not go on to say that the procedure will probably make the contractions more painful.

Midwives are sometimes selective in the information that they give to women. Kirkham noted that the midwife's decision whether or not to give information was made, in part, on the woman's perceived social class (remember social attribution?) Women who were seen to be 'intelligent' or of a higher social class were more likely to be perceived as 'nice' and to receive answers to questions. Women who were seen to be from a lower social class were often denied information. This may also be true of other aspects of maternity care. Hemingway *et al* (1997) found that women who spoke English and were from social classes I–III were more likely to receive continuity of care. Such a strategy is entirely unacceptable, because as we pointed out in earlier chapters, a midwife's assessment of an individual's ability to understand information may well be based on her own subjective stereotypes and prejudices.

All women are familiar with their own bodies and will state, in their own words or actions, what they are feeling. The midwife needs to respect this knowledge and to develop excellent communication skills in order to understand the text and the sub-text of what is being said. This requires perception on the part of the midwife to understand both verbal and non-verbal communication, such as tone of voice and body posture. Open, ongoing and honest communication is an essential facet of individualised care that can enhance women's birth experiences. If communication is excellent women will retain a sense of control, dignity and power whether or not the birth turns out as they had planned. A breakdown in communication can leave women with memories that cause them acute distress for many years (Simkin, 1991). It seems likely that poor communication might become a particular problem if complications develop during labour. When there is an acute sense of urgency the midwife has to deal with her own anxieties and concerns. The need for good communication never diminishes and it is when women are feeling most vulnerable that they will need to understand not only what is happening, but why this is so.

When things go differently

Although most women expect to have an uncomplicated birth, there are always some instances when things do not go according to plan; a small percentage will need medical intervention in the form of an operative or instrumental delivery and this does not take into account the number of women who have more 'minor' intervention, such as augmentation of labour. Large numbers of women do not have the type of birth they might have planned or wished for. What is the effect of this clash between hope and reality? Joan Raphael-Leff (1993) suggests that women who require a Caesarean section may feel cheated of the birth that they had planned, may blame themselves for not giving birth 'normally' and may feel angry and violated by the experience. One woman, interviewed by another author, describes her acute feelings of loss and diminished self-esteem:

Very little seems to be written about the psychological effect a Caesarean can have upon a woman — guilt, anxiety and failure. The experience shattered me and my confidence in myself as a woman and gave me a feeling of

failure at not being able to perform the function for which
I, as a woman, was intended — having a baby...

(Kitzinger, 1987, p.113)

Research by Trowell (1982) also demonstrates that mothers who require an emergency Caesarean section may experience long-term feelings of failure as a woman, and resentment towards the baby for not 'coming out'.

Oakley and Richards (1990) comment on the use of the term 'section' rather than operation or surgery to describe a Caesarean. As a result, the psychological consequences of major surgery, such as depression, may not be acknowledged or recognised (for further exploration of these themes, see *Chapter 9*).

Research by Green *et al* (1998) found that women who had a Caesarean section that was 'elective' and was planned well in advance were more satisfied than those who had an emergency Caesarean. Perhaps more surprisingly, their research also showed that women who required intervention in labour were not automatically concerned about the procedure itself, but by its perceived necessity. This brings us back to the issue of communication, and the importance of clear, honest information that enables women to know not only what is happening but why. Women who understand the necessity of an intervention, however major or minor, are far less likely to experience adverse psychological consequences.

Raphael-Leff (1993) points out that feelings of loss and failure are not unique to women who have had a Caesarean, but may also be detected in women who have experienced unanticipated problems. Women who have a long and difficult labour may regret the 'perfect birth' they had anticipated. Similarly, a short labour may be equally traumatic and shocking: the woman who has a short labour will probably be given less sympathy, and told that she is lucky. Women whose baby is born prematurely or requires resuscitation; women planning a home birth who have to be transferred to hospital; women who require an instrumental delivery, or an epidural having hoped to avoid pharmacological analgesia may all feel that the birth has gone 'differently'. The skill of the midwife lies in ensuring that women understand what happened and why. The study by Berg and Dahlberg (1998) demonstrated that women could feel very positive about their birth experience even when they developed complications in labour. Women attribute these positive feelings to the support and individualised care that they received from the midwife. The provision of good support from chosen birth companions and from the midwife, underpinned by excellent communication, may prevent a potentially adverse event being remembered in completely negative terms. In an ideal world, all women would remember their birth experiences with affection and pride. While this might not be possible, good midwifery support can ensure that when things go differently women do not blame themselves and are not left mulling over unanswered questions.

Post-traumatic stress disorder and labour

Post-traumatic stress disorder (PTSD) was first defined almost twenty years ago (Lyons, 1998), although it is only in more recent years that the condition has been discussed in particular relation to midwifery care. The American Psychiatric Association (1994) describes PTSD as:

> *The re-experiencing of an extremely traumatic event accompanied by symptoms of increased arousal and by avoidance of stimuli associated with the traumata.*

(p. 393)

In simpler terms, this means that a person who has experienced a traumatic event will continue to relive that event and may experience upsetting flashbacks which are both vivid and disturbing. However, the individual will, where possible, take steps to try and avoid reminders of the trauma. Despite this avoidance there may still be an awareness of changes in behaviour, sensitivity to arousal, sleep disturbances and mood swings. Given that some women have difficult births, which they experience as traumatic, it seems perfectly possible that women may suffer from PTSD after giving birth.

One factor that may be crucial in the prevention of PTSD is a woman's sense of control (Lyons, 1998). As was discussed earlier in this chapter, Green *et al* (1998) have shown that women who have a potentially traumatic birth, with lots of intervention, can be satisfied with their birth experience if they felt that they had some control over the intervention. It cannot be assumed that women who have an intervention-free-birth will not experience PTSD. Crompton (1996) points out that childbirth may re-traumatise survivors of previous trauma. One area of increasing awareness is that birth may remind women of previous sexual abuse (Kirkman, 1998).

One possible remedy that may be offered to women who have had a traumatic birth, in the hope of voiding PTSD is a debriefing service. Raphael-Leff (1993) argues that all women should be offered the opportunity to meet with their midwife a day or two after the birth for what she describes as a 'debriefing chat' (p. 122). In an attempt to improve services to women and to provide more effective risk management, some health authorities have implemented a debriefing service (Smith and Mitchell, 1996). Some authors (Kirkham *et al*, 1997) have expressed concern about the implementation of formal debriefing services, and call for a randomised controlled trial to demonstrate its effectiveness. They differentiate between the 'debriefing chat' described by Raphael-Leff which, they suggest, midwives have probably always done, and the more structured and formal service that is now available in some areas. Kirkham *et al* point out that it is not sufficient to implement a new form of practice such as debriefing simply because it seems harmless and sounds as though it should be a good idea.

Recent evidence suggests that debriefing needs to be viewed with some caution. Small *et al* (2000) conducted a randomised controlled trial of midwife-led debriefing. The participants were 1041 women who had given birth by Caesarean section or with the use of forceps or vacuum extraction. Half the women received debriefing and half did not. Results indicated that more women who had received debriefing were depressed six months later than those who had not, although 43% of women rated the debriefing session as 'very helpful' and 51% as 'helpful'. It would appear from this study that debriefing may not be a universal panacea for women who have experienced a 'traumatic birth'.

Some women in the study by Garcia *et al* (1998) stated that they wished that they had had the opportunity to talk through the experience afterwards, in order to clarify for themselves what had happened and why. It is hard to know what is the real difference between this and a formal debriefing service, although the latter is available in the longer term. Smith and Mitchell (1996) comment that the women using their service had had their babies between four weeks and forty-five years previously. Lyons (1998) suggests that there are occasions when debriefing by the midwife present at the birth, whether in an informal or more structured capacity, may not be helpful, particularly if the woman feels angry or antagonistic towards the midwife concerned. There are situations in which a trained counsellor may be used as a mediator to enable the woman and midwife to meet in a more constructive and less hostile atmosphere.

Whatever the continuing debates about debriefing show in the future, the prevention of PTSD is the most important goal. The provision of sensitive, midwifery care, which enables women to feel a sense of control over the birth experience, may in the long run be more effective than formal debriefing services.

Childbirth preparation

How do women prepare for the experience of labour? They may wish to listen to reports from family members and friends, but they may be exposed to such reports even if they would prefer not to. They will be exposed to media information in magazines designed for that purpose, in newspapers which may be highlighting the most recent 'scare stories', and on television, both 'soaps' and documentaries. The affect of all these influences will not be discussed in detail, but just serve as a reminder that there are many influences from a woman's social environment and culture that will influence her expectations of labour and birth. It is worth pointing out the results of a piece of research that demonstrated the discrepancy between portrayals of childbirth on television and the reality of birth (Clement, 1997). This study revealed that, on television, birth is depicted as fast, unpredictable, drug-free, and dangerous. Clement's work also notes that, on average, one birth is shown on British television every four days. With such constant bombardment of inaccurate information, is it any wonder that many women and their partners attend the hospital very early in labour. They must be acutely anxious about the birth and an off-hand comment by the midwife along the lines of, 'Oh, you've got hours to go yet' will do little to allay these fears.

In an attempt to gain more accurate and specific information, some women will attend childbirth preparation classes, either those provided by the hospital, or those organised by a lay association such as the National Childbirth Trust. (I am aware that there is a lot of discussion about what these sessions should be called. Some people dislike the term 'classes' finding it reminiscent of school and therefore potentially alienating to some women. In order not to get embroiled into semantic arguments I will use the terms 'classes' and 'childbirth preparation classes' interchangeably — clumsy, but descriptive.)

One of the stated purposes of many childbirth preparation classes is to teach women breathing exercises and coping strategies. The classes also usually attempt to give women information about the birth process so that they have a clearer idea of the signs of labour, and of some of the physical and emotional sensations they may experience. (Having said this, I am aware that many classes now do not have a formal agenda and claim to be 'led by the women' so that the women decide for themselves what subjects will be covered in each session. Nevertheless, I assert that most classes will have similar content. It is the way and the order in which this content is discussed that may vary more widely.)

One author (Niven, 1992) has suggested that there are two ways in which women respond to information about labour and birth. Niven describes those women who do not actively seek information as 'deniers' and implies that such women may ignore or deny what they are told, while the 'vigilant' person wants detailed information. Niven goes on to suggest that deniers are less likely to go to classes. I do not find these classifications particularly helpful. A midwife who has decided that someone is a 'denier' may then think it is reasonable to withhold information from her, as she would ignore it. It is important, however, that the midwife asks the woman whether or not she wants information. This may seem to be stating the obvious but perhaps there is no harm in that. All women are entitled to full and detailed information if that is what they want, but some women, for whatever reasons, may not want this. Midwives need to be aware of women's individual wishes and be flexible in their approach. Niven also discusses the need to give women 'sensory information' about the birth process. She defines this as the description of the sights, sounds, smells, tastes and tactile experiences of birth, in a language that women can understand. Niven suggests that this will avoid the problem of women saying, 'But no-one told me what it would be really like'. I am not convinced of the benefits of this, but is this just my squeamishness in not wanting to discuss the possible intensity of labour pain? I think that the debate as to the benefits of sensory information merit further study.

It has been suggested that the aim of childbirth preparation classes is to address concerns of anxiety and pain and also to provide information-giving (Niven, 1992). There is little evidence that classes are successful in alleviating anxiety (Astbury, 1980; Brewin and Bradley, 1982). Similarly, Green *et al*'s study (1998) indicated that women who were anxious about the pain of labour were more likely to have a negative birth experience. This does not mean that classes are unsuccessful but perhaps that the focus of childbirth preparation should be on providing women with coping strategies to deal with their anxiety. It would be unrealistic to expect that midwives can allay all anxieties, some of which will be very deep-seated, but they can attempt to reassure women that such anxieties are normal.

Giving women a chance to express these anxieties is important in itself: in acknowledging them they can begin to deal with them.

The results of the 'Great Expectations' research (Green *et al*, 1998) have shown that women tend to experience what they expected in labour and birth. The women who had the lowest expectations in the study were also the most likely to report dissatisfaction with their birth experience. This would suggest that one way in which classes might benefit women is by providing them with information which might (and I stress might) increase their expectations. It is said that 'knowledge is power'. I would argue that this is not true in every circumstance but knowledge certainly gives greater potential for power. Green *et al*'s study concluded that a perceived sense of control is the most important factor in enabling women to have a positive birth experience.

Discussions about the effectiveness of childbirth preparation classes continue. As Niven (1992) has pointed out, many women do not find that classes meet their expectations. One of the obvious problems is that each individual within a group attending the same class will have a different agenda. Even couples who have attended the class together will hope for information tailored to their unique needs. I had a recent experience of this chatting to a woman who had been very disappointed in the classes she attended. What she had wanted was to be taught how to bath a baby. Antenatal classes are based on the assumption that women 'need' information about labour and childbirth but it is possibly rather unrealistic to think that classes can provide for all these unique needs. Again, I do not wish to suggest that women should be denied information but I wonder whether classes are the best forum for this sort of information-giving.

Conclusion

As Sherr (1995) points out, the emphasis on women's emotional and psychological needs in childbirth is a relatively recent phenomenon:

> *In the early days... the overriding issue of mortality and morbidity demanded most attention [and] there was little focus on the emotional well being of the mother, let alone her wider family.*

> (p. 208)

In the Western world at the beginning of the twenty-first century we are fortunate in having relatively low rates of both maternal and perinatal mortality and morbidity. Of course, the relative physical safety of the mother and baby are of paramount importance but this does not mean that psychological care in labour is a luxury. As I stated at the beginning of the chapter, women may remember their birth experiences for the rest of their lives. As a midwife you are in the privileged position of witnessing that experience. It may not be possible to give all women 'the perfect birth' but I hope that, having read this chapter, you will have a clearer awareness of some of the complex factors involved.

The key to all of this is flexibility. If you can be flexible in your approach to each woman you care for, you are in a position to respond to her particular needs. All the different issues that have been discussed, such as pain and anxiety in labour, and the role of birth companions are vitally important. Each birth that you attend as a midwife will be different; there may be many common factors between them, but nonetheless each one is unique. A deeper understanding of some of the psychological issues that might have an impact on a woman in labour will enhance your practice.

References

Alexander J (1998) Confusing debriefing and refusing postnatally: the need for clarity of terms, purpose and value. *Midwifery* **14**(2): 122–4

American Psychiatric Association (1994) *Diagnostic and statistical manual of mental disorders.* 4th edn. APA, Washington DC

Astbury J (1980) Labour pain: the role of childbirth education, information and education. In: Peck C, Wallace M, eds. *Problems in Pain.* Pergamon, London

Berg M, Lundgren I, Hermansson E *et al* (1996) Women's experience of the encounter with the midwife during childbirth. *Midwifery* **12**(1): 11–15

Berg M, Dahlberg K (1998) A phenomenological study of women's experiences of complicated childbirth. *Midwifery* **14**(1): 23–9

Bluff R, Holloway I (1994) They know best: women's perceptions of midwifery care during labour and childbirth. *Midwifery* **10**(3): 157–64

Brewin C, Bradley C (1982) Perceived control and the experience of childbirth. *Br J Clin Psychol* **21**: 263–9

Budden S (1998) Eleanor's birth. *Midwifery Matters* **77**: 14–7

Capogna G, Alahuhta S, Celleno D, De Vlieger H, Moreira J, Morgan B *et al* (1996) Maternal expectations and experiences of labour pain: a multi-centre study of nulliparous women. *Int J Obstet Anesthesia* **5**(4): 229–35

Clement S (1997) Childbirth on television. *Br J Midwifery* **5**(1): 37–42

Crafter H (2000) Psychology of pain in normal labour. In: Yerby M, ed. *Pain in Childbearing: Key issues in management.* Baillière Tindall, London

Department of Health (1993) *Changing Childbirth: Report of the Expert Maternity Group.* HMSO, London

Garcia J, Garforth S (1990) Parents and new-born babies in the labour ward. In: Garcia J, Kilpatrick R, Richards M, eds. *The Politics of Maternity Care: Services for Childbearing Women in Twentieth-Century Britain.* Clarendon Press, Oxford

Garcia J, Redshaw M, Fitzsimmons B, Keene J (1998) *First Class Delivery: a National Survey of Women's Views on Maternity Care.* Audit Commission, London

Green J M, Coupland VA, Kitzinger JV (1998) *Great Expectations: a Prospective Study of Women's Expectations and Experiences of Childbirth.* Books for Midwives Press, Hale

Halldorsdottir S, Karlsdottir SI (1996) Journeying through labour and delivery: perceptions of women who have given birth. *Midwifery* 12(2): 48–61

Hemingway H, Saunders D, parsons L (1997) Social class, spoken language and pattern of care as determinants of continuity of carer in maternity services in east London. *J Public Health Med* 19(2): 156–61

Hodnett ED (2000) *Caregiver support for women during childbirth.* Cochrane Database System Review (2): CD000199

Hundley VA, Milne JM, Glazener CM, Mollison J (1997) Satisfaction and the three 'Cs': continuity, choice and control. Women's views from a randomised controlled trial of midwife-led care. *Br J Obstet Gynaecol* 104(119): 1273–80

Hunt S, Symonds A (1994) *The Social Meaning of Midwifery.* Macmillan Press, Basingstoke

Illich I (1976) *Limits to Medicine. Medical Nemesis: the Expropriation of Health.* Penguin, London

Jackson K (1996) It's only words. *Br J Midwifery* 4(12): 665

Katbamna S (2000) *Race and Childbirth.* Open University Press, Buckingham

Kennell J, Klaus M, McGrath S, Robertson S, Kinkley C (1991) Continuous emotional support during labour in a US hospital. A randomized controlled trial. *JAMA* 265(17): 2197–201

Kirkham S (1989) Midwives and information-giving during labour. In: Robinson S, Thomson AM, eds. *Midwives, Research and Childbirth.* Vol 1. Chapman and Hall, London

Kirkham M, Garcia J, Alexander J (1997) Debriefing after childbirth (correspondence). *Br J Midwifery* 5(2): 74

Kirkman S (1998) The emotional pain of labour. *MIDIRS Midwifery Digest* 8(3): 328–30

Kitzinger S (1978) Pain in childbirth. *J Med Ethics* 4: 119–21

Kitzinger S (1987) *Giving Birth: How it Really Feels.* Gollancz, London

Klaus MH, Kennell JH (1997) The doula: an essential ingredient of childbirth rediscovered. *Acta Paediatr* 86(10): 1034–6

Lowe NK (1996) The pain and discomfort of labour and birth. *J Obstet Gynecol Neonatal Nurs* 25(1): 82–92

Lyons S (1998) Post-traumatic stress disorder following childbirth: causes, prevention and treatment. In: Clement S, ed. *Psychological Perspectives on Pregnancy and Childbirth*. Churchill Livingstone, Edinburgh

Macdonald KM (1995) *The Sociology of the Professions*. Sage Publications, London

Mander R (1998) *Pain in Childbirth and its Control*. Blackwell Science, Oxford

McCrea BH, Wright ME (1999) Satisfaction in childbirth and perception of personal control in labour. *J Adv Nurs* **29**(4): 877–84.

McCrea H, Wright ME, Stringer M (2000) Psychosocial factors influencing personal control in pain relief. *Int J Nurs Stud* **37**(6): 493–503

Melzack R, Wall PD (1965) Pain mechanisms: A new theory. *Science* **150**(4): 971–9.

Melzack R, Wall PD (1998) *The Challenge of Pain*. Penguin, Harmondsworth

Moore S (1994) Pain relief in labour: an overview. *Br J Midwifery* **2**(10): 483–6

Moore S (1997) Psychology of pain in labour. In: Moore S, ed. *Understanding Pain and its Relief in Labour*. Churchill Livingstone, New York

Niven CA (1992) *Psychological Care for Families: Before, During and After Birth*. Butterworth Heinemann, Oxford

Niven C (1994) Coping with labour pain; the midwife's role. In: Robinson S, Thomson AM, eds. *Midwives, Research and Childbirth*. Vol 3. Chapman and Hall, London

Oakley A, Richards M (1990) Women's experiences of Caesarean delivery. In: Garcia J, Kilpatrick R, Richards M, eds. *The Politics of Maternity Care: Services for Childbearing Women in Twentieth Century Britain*. Clarendon Press, Oxford

O'Driscoll K, Meagher D (1980) *Active Management of Labour*. Baillière Tindall, London

Olsen O (1997) Meta-analysis of the safety of home birth. *Birth* **24**(1): 4–13

Page LA, Vail A, Beake S (1996) Results of the clinical audit. In: McCourt C, Page L, eds. *Report on the Evaluation of One-to One Midwifery*. Thames Valley University, London

Pollard J, Robotham M (1998) Midwife-led units: the heat is on. *MIDIRS Midwifery Digest* **8**(2): 150–1

Price J (1988) *Motherhood: What It Does To Your Mind*. Pandora, London

Price S (1998) Birth plans and their impact on midwifery care. *MIDIRS Midwifery Digest* **8**(2): 189–91

Raphael-Leff J (1991) *Psychological Processes of Childbearing*. Chapman and Hall, London

Raphael-Leff J (1993) *Pregnancy: The inside story*. Sheldon Press, London

Rogers J (1998) Birth plans (correspondence). *Br J Midwifery* **6**(8): 524

Schott J, Henley A (1996) *Culture, Religion and Childbearing in a Multi-racial Society: a Handbook for Health Professionals*. Butterworth-Heinemann, Oxford

Sheiner EK, Sheiner E, Shoham-Vardi I, Mazor M, Katz M (1999) Ethnic differences influence care giver's estimates of pain during labour. *Pain* **81**(3) 299–305

Sherr L (1995) *The Psychology of Pregnancy and Childbirth*. Blackwell Science, Oxford

Simkin P (1991) Just another day in a woman's life? Women's long-term perceptions of their first birth experience. *Birth* **18**(4): 203–10

Small R, Lumley J, Donohue L, Potter A, Waldenström U (2000) Randomised controlled trial of midwife-led debriefing to reduce maternal depression after operative childbirth. *Br Med J* **321**: 1043–7

Smith JA, Mitchell S (1996) Debriefing after childbirth: a tool for effective risk management. *Br J Midwifery* **4**(11): 581–6

Squire C (2000) Sociocultural aspects of pain. In: Yerby M, ed. *Pain in Childbearing: Key issues in management.* Baillière Tindall, London

Symonds A, Hunt SC (1996) *The Midwife and Society: Perspectives, Policies and Practice.* Macmillan Press Ltd, Basingstoke

Taylor K, Copstick S (1985) Psychological care in labour. *Nurs Mirror* **161**(4): 42–3

Trowell J (1982) Possible effects of emergency Caesarean section on mother-child relationship. *Early Hum Dev* **7**: 41–51

United Kingdom Central Council for Nursing, Midwifery and Health Visiting (1993) *Midwives Rules.* UKCC, London

United Kingdom Central Council for Nursing, Midwifery and Health Visiting (1994) *The Midwives Code of Practice.* UKCC, London

Waldenstrom U, Turnbull D (1998) A systematic review comparing continuity of midwifery care with standard maternity services. *Br J Obstet Gynaecol* **105**(11): 1160–70

Weaver J (1998) Choice, control and decision-making in labour. In: Clement S, ed. *Psychological Perspectives on Pregnancy and Childbirth.* Churchill Livingstone, Edinburgh

Yerby M (1996) Managing pain in labour. *Modern Midwife* **6**(3): 22–4

Yerby M, ed (2000) *Pain in Childbearing: Key issues in management.* Baillière Tindall, London

8

Early infancy: what can the newborn do?

The birth of a new baby always seems miraculous and as a midwife you are privileged to be part of this momentous life event almost every day of your working life, but once the baby has been safely delivered and pronounced healthy, what is she capable of? Is she simply a rather blotchy bundle of wriggling, crying flesh totally unprepared for the complexity of the world into which she has been precipitated, or is there something more? Until relatively recently it was thought that babies do indeed come into the world with almost no innate abilities; it was commonly believed that babies, like puppies and kittens, were blind at birth. Infants were considered to be totally helpless with little genetically pre-programmed behaviours to enable them to survive. However, at the beginning of the twenty-first century, we have a very different picture of the newborn. We are now reasonably sure that they are equipped from birth with many abilities that help them to begin to make sense of their physical environment and form relationships with those who care for them.

Although the midwife does not spend long with the new baby, it is important for her to have some understanding of the psychological capacities of infants in the early days of life. The early mother/infant relationship is complex and what happens in the first days may have an impact on later development. Because the midwife is the health professional who cares for the mother and baby at the very beginning of their relationship, it is possible that she can have a positive impact, by helping the mother to understand what her baby is capable of and what his needs are.

This chapter first considers the perceptual and social abilities of the newborn, and then goes on to explore aspects of the infant's relationship with his or her primary caregivers. For the majority of time, I will confine the discussion to the very early days of life, but at times it may be necessary to look at the slightly older baby, to give a fuller understanding of what exactly is developing.

How do we study infants?

Developmental textbooks frequently quote a statement that was made by William James, one of the first psychologists. He believed that the newborn must experience the world as chaotic and disorganised. In his words:

> *The baby assailed by ears, nose, skin and entrails at once, feels it all one great blooming, buzzing confusion.*

> ([1890 p. 488] quoted in McShane, 1991 p. 43)

Although this view of infancy was held for many decades, we now know that this is not really an accurate picture, babies do seem to be able to organise the environmental stimuli that must hit them when they arrive in the world. Before we talk in more detail about the abilities of the newborn it is important to discuss first how psychologists have gone about finding out what infants can do.

As you can probably imagine, tiny babies are not at all easy to study. To begin with, they do not really do very much apart from eat, sleep and cry and the times when they are awake and fully alert are rather limited. In order to study their abilities they do need to be in this alert, wakeful state. The second difficulty is that infants cannot tell you what they are experiencing because they have not yet acquired language. Psychologists have to infer this from other aspects of the infant's behaviour that can be observed. However, undaunted by these limitations and with the help of ingenious research techniques and modern technology, we are gradually building up a picture of the perceptual capacities of the newborn.

The oldest and most basic and useful research technique is observation. We have learned a great deal about infant behaviour from careful and detailed observation of the newborn. While careful and accurate observation is an essential part of any experimental technique, in order to understand more complex behaviour we need methods that enable us to theorise what might be going on in the brain of the neonate. Fantz (1961) was one of the earliest researchers to look at the visual capacities of the infant and he invented a technique for studying this called preferential looking. His method was extremely simple but effective. He reasoned that if a baby is given a choice of two things to look at and spends longer looking at one than the other, then it is reasonable to assume that the baby finds the object that he looks at longest more interesting. A fairly simple research apparatus was designed in which an observer could look down on the infant and note which of two stimuli presented at the same time the infant looked at longest.

Other researchers have found habituation to be helpful when looking at infant behaviour. We have all experienced habituation occurring in our day-to-day lives. It is what happens when you no longer notice the sound of a clock ticking in a room, even though it might have appeared quite loud when you first entered the room. If you have a pet at home you can test out habituation for yourself. If you make a loud noise such as clapping your hands, your dog or cat (or even the hamster) will show a startled response to the sound. Pavlov called this the orienting reflex (Pavlov, 1927 quoted in McShane, 1991). If you then wait for the animal to settle down and repeat the noise, they will show a startled response again, but this time they will not react as much. If you repeat this process several times the animal will eventually ignore the noise completely. In other words they have habituated to the unusual sound. However, if you change the noise in some way, the orienting reflex will re-emerge.

Just like human adults and animals, babies demonstrate the habituation response and it has been used to study many aspects of infant ability including learning, memory, perceptual discrimination and categorisation (McShane, 1991). The technique involves two stages. In the initial phase the baby is shown a stimulus until they no longer attend to it (one might suggest that the baby has become bored with it), once this point has been reached the stimulus is changed slightly. If the attention of the baby returns on presentation of the new, novel stimulus, one can reasonably assume that they are able to perceive the difference between the first stimulus and the second. If the baby does not show any interest in the second stimulus then the researcher may conclude that the infant perceives the two stimuli as the same and cannot perceive differences between them.

A third method involves using physiological responses such as heart rate and EEG patterns. These measurements reflect the level of physiological arousal. As McShane (1991, p. 46) points out:

Changes in level of arousal indicate changes in the processing of environmental information. When an organism detects novel or significant environmental events a number of changes are triggered by the autonomic nervous system, which include changes in heart rate, sweat gland activity, pupil dilation and EEG activity. These changes can be monitored and used as indirect measures of the detection and selection of information in the environment.

Heart rate is the physiological measure that has been used most frequently and it can either accelerate or decelerate from a previously measured baseline. Some researchers have argued that a deceleration occurs when infants are aroused because they are interested in a novel event, acceleration of heart rate occurs when infants are alarmed by an event. But there is some dispute about this.

We have four techniques that have been used to find out what infants are capable of. These techniques, coupled with powerful computers and video, have enabled us to discover much about the human infant. However, as always in psychology, difficulties remain which must make us cautious in the interpretation of results. When discussing infant abilities we must always be clear that by observing behaviour we can only ever infer what is going on in the infant's mind. There is always the possibility that our inferences, however reasonable they seem, could be wrong. Such caution is warranted when one considers that it has not always been possible to repeat results when studies have been replicated and different methods have also produced different results. Bearing these comments in mind, let us consider the research findings in more detail.

What can the newborn do?

Reflexes

Every infant is born with a set of readily observable reflexes, some of which still exist in the adult and will be familiar to you, such as the knee jerk reflex, the eye blink reflex, and the contraction of the pupil when in bright light. Other infant reflexes are controlled by the primitive midbrain and gradually diminish as the baby develops. Some of these, nevertheless, are extremely important for survival. The rooting reflex which causes the infant to turn in the direction of a stroke on the cheek and the sucking reflex are both crucial for feeding and sustaining life, as is the breathing reflex.

The life-sustaining functions of some of the other reflexes are less easy to understand. These include the moro reflex (the infant throws out her arms and legs and arches her back when she hears a loud noise or anything else that startles her), the Babinsky reflex (the infant curls his toes around an object pressed into the ball of the foot), and the grasp reflex (the infant grasps tightly any object placed in the palm of the hand). Infants also show the stepping reflex. If they are held in an upright position with their feet on a flat surface, they will then make walking movements. It is hard to understand exactly the purpose of these reflexes, one can only presume that they are the remnants of behaviour that had survival value in our evolutionary past. Another explanation for the stepping reflex suggests that it has been learned by the fetus while in utero in order to turn around (Bremner 1994). This is certainly an intriguing possibility and appears to be a logical explanation for behaviour that is otherwise difficult to understand. Unfortunately, some of the other reflexes do not seem to have such a meaningful explanation of their origin and purpose.

Regardless of their origins, reflexes are important at birth and can be an indication of the health of the baby. They may be significant in other ways too. Jean Piaget believed that infant reflexes were the building blocks for all other aspects of cognitive development.

The simple reflexes with which the neonate is endowed soon undergo definite modifications as a consequence of environmental contact; in so doing they imperceptibly become acquired adaptations instead of mere reflexes.

(Flavell, 1963, p. 89)

Sleeping and waking states

Babies differ in their levels of wakefulness from birth. Initially, they may be drowsy and unresponsive because the mother has received medication; although there is some debate about the long-term effects of drugs like pethidine, the short-term effects seem to quickly wear off. Newborn infants then seem to dip in and out of different levels of arousal. Some authors have regarded these as different points on a continuum, while others see them as discreet states.

The levels of arousal have been described as deep sleep, active sleep, quiet awake, active awake and crying and fussing. On average, at birth, the infant will spend up to eighteen hours in every twenty-four asleep, and the remainder in one or other of the wakeful states. Of course, there are enormous individual differences and some parents may be forgiven for thinking that their new baby never sleeps but simply cries all the time.

Sadly, new babies do not come into the world knowing the difference between night and day and their wakeful periods may occur at times when their parents would much prefer them to be asleep. This can have some impact on the parent/child relationship.

Temperament

Certain gross temperamental differences appear to be apparent from birth and may even have their origins before birth (Eaton and Saudino, 1992). These temperamental differences appear to be quite stable over the first few months of life and do not seem to be related to the way babies are treated by their parents (Bremner, 1994). Back in 1977 Thomas and Chess described three types of infant temperament that have been used subsequently in other studies. They suggested that babies could be classified as easy, difficult, and slow to warm up.

❖ The easy child seems to approach most new events positively, they have regular biological habits, eating, sleeping, eliminating and adjust easily to change. The kind of baby everyone would like.

❖ The difficult child is the opposite of the easy child. She tends to react negatively to anything new, cries more and is not regular in biological habits. A baby with this kind of disposition will take longer to develop regular routines and is generally harder to handle.

❖ The slow to warm up child just seems to show a kind of passive resistance. They react both more positively and more negatively to new events, but eventually seem to settle down in a positive way.

❖ There was a fourth group too, which consisted of those infants who did not appear to fit any of the three categories described above.

So far, there is only scant evidence that such temperament differences are directly linked to subsequent personality (Stratton, 1982). Izard *et al* (2000) have argued that emotional variables measured in babies can predict temperament up to the age of two years and Fox and Henderson (1999) suggest that elements of infant temperament predict social behaviour in the pre-school period. Of course, the temperament of the baby and the way it is perceived by the parents will inevitably influence the way the parents handle her. This may indirectly have an impact on later behaviour but this will also depend on a variety of other factors, such as the relationship between the parents. A complex range of variables will influence the developing child and clearly further research is needed in this area before firm conclusions can be drawn about the relationship between infant temperament and later behaviour.

There is some evidence that there are cultural differences in infant temperament.

Signalling emotional states: crying and smiling

Probably the first thing that most newborn babies do is cry. It is the only way that the newborn has of signalling negative emotional states and although initially it is not a learned behaviour, the infant very quickly learns that crying can be used as an effective form of communication.

From the beginning, there appear to be three categories of cry that signal different states in the baby. These were first recorded and described by Wolff (1969). The basic cry is often a response to hunger and consists of a cry lasting about 0.6 seconds, followed by a brief pause of about 0.2 seconds, a sharp intake of breath, which lasts between 0.1. and 0.2 seconds and then another pause before the next cry. The angry cry is similar to the basic cry, but there are shorter pauses between the cries. The third type of cry is the pain cry. Of the three types of cry this is the hardest for adults to ignore. Wolff recorded this when infants were having blood samples taken from the heel and it consists of a loud wail followed by a prolonged period of breath holding. Of course, not all cries fit exactly into these three groups, but consist of variations of all three.

Perhaps the most important aspect of the infant cry is the effect it has on adults. Few can listen for long without doing something. Although there is some variation in the way people respond, the infant cry appears to have an arousing effect on the listener. It is not clear exactly why we find the sound of an infant crying so distressing, but adults do seem to be motivated to stop the crying as quickly as possible. Usually the adult assumes that the infant intends to communicate something by the cry and will make efforts to discover what is causing the problem. This can lead to parental frustration when everything has been tried and yet the infant continues to cry. In some cases, this can lead to tragic consequences.

Although not necessarily apparent at birth, smiling is another aspect of the infants' behavioural repertoire that communicates emotional states to the adult caregivers. There is some disagreement about the onset of smiling behaviour and whether it is initially social or not. However, something that looks like a smile or what has been described rather technically as 'Bilateral extensions of the outer lip' have been observed in neonates and even in utero (Durkin, 1995, p. 47). Perhaps as Trevarthen (1982) maintains, we are missing the point when we wrangle over whether the basis of the smile is physiological or social. The important thing is that a smile only has meaning within a social context and it has a profound impact on those who observe it.

Who can resist that gummy, toothless grin? It is a hard-hearted person indeed who does not smile back and encourage the baby to try to elicit another smile. Like crying, over a period of months the baby quickly learns to use the smile to engage in social interaction, and adults respond by talking and playing with the baby.

Taken together, crying and smiling provide two essential signals to the adult caregiver. The cry demonstrating discomfort and the need for a change in the current state of things, the smile showing that the baby is enjoying what is happening. As Durkin states:

> *The cry conveys the message, 'come and sort this out' while the smile relays 'that's good, do it again'. The infant is biologically equipped to signal its states in patterned ways which mature members of the species can interpret reasonably well — and the mature members of the species are biologically disposed to react to the stimuli the infant provides.*

> (1995, p. 50)

Vision

What can the newborn see? The short answer to this question is that while the baby cannot see as well as a baby of six months or an adult, their visual system is sufficiently well formed for them to be able to focus on a near object (about eight inches seems to be optimal). Both eyes work well together so that by a few weeks old the infant can track a moving object and by one month can discriminate their mother's face from others (Bee, 1992). In terms of survival, this degree of visual capacity is adequate. The baby does not really need to be able to see objects at great distances as they spend much of their time asleep and, in the feeding situation, their ability to focus on a point at about eight inches means that they can see their mother's face quite well. Various aspects of infant visual perception have been studied in more detail. From these a picture emerges of a system that is somewhat immature but which rapidly develops to function as well as the adult. Visual accommodation refers to the ability to focus on a distant object. At birth, this ability is limited so the newborn has some difficulty focusing, but by four months visual accommodation is similar to the adult. In general, infants under a month old find it easier to accommodate to a near object rather than one at a distance.

Visual acuity is the ability to discriminate fine detail.

Traditionally this has been measured using diagrams of vertical stripes, the thickness of which is gradually reduced until the visual system is no longer able to differentiate the stripes which blur into each other so that the diagram appears a uniform grey. At about two weeks the stripes on such diagrams have to be thirty times wider apart than they would have to be for an adult for the baby to be able to recognise that they are stripes. By six months they only have to be ten times wider apart. What this means is that the baby finds it difficult to discriminate fine detail. I often think for the baby it must be like being short-sighted (if you are you know what I mean) when you take your glasses off everything beyond a certain distance appears in a blur. If you are not short-sighted and find this hard to imagine, just think what objects would look like to you if you were seeing them through a pane of frosted glass.

As well as acuity or fine discrimination, the adult is also sensitive to contrasts between light and shade. This ability is obviously important in allowing us to discriminate objects in our environment. Once again, we find that the infant's visual system is not as good at this as the adult but improvement is rapid, particularly in the first six months of life.

We also know that infants appear to be attracted to patterns, they seem to like to look at them. Fantz (1961) who we have already mentioned, showed that even newborns show reliable preferences for certain kinds of patterns. Initially newborns seem to prefer less complex patterns, for example 2 x 2 squares on a checkerboard, but gradually as the infant gets older, they like more and more complex visual stimuli. They also seem to be attracted to patterns with high contrast. The explanation for this could be that such patterns help to exercise the visual system and provide the necessary stimuli for it to develop.

A lot of research has been devoted to the infant's perception of depth. However, due to methodological problems it is difficult to demonstrate this in children under three or four months of age, so we do not know whether or not the newborn is able to perceive depth or whether some interaction with the environment is necessary for this to develop. We do know that newborns possess shape constancy; that is, the ability to recognise that an object is the same shape even when it is tilted and casts a different image on the retina (Slater and Morison, 1985). Size constancy, or the ability to know that an object is the same size regardless of whether it is near or further away, has not yet been demonstrated in neonates.

This is only a very brief summary of our current state of knowledge about the infant's visual system (for a more detailed but accessible account see McShane, 1991). What it shows, I believe, is that from birth the baby can use vision to acquire a great deal of information about its environment. It has been claimed that the system is set up biologically to extract the optimum amount of information for development to occur. Whether this is ultimately found to be true or not I think it is helpful for mothers and midwives to have an understanding of the infant's visual capabilities. To know that the baby can clearly see the mother's face while feeding must surely encourage the mother to gaze at her baby and talk to him, which will undoubtedly aid the development of their relationship. An understanding that the baby will enjoy looking at simple objects and patterns should also encourage the parents to provide such stimuli and to play with the baby during periods of wakefulness. This kind of play not only helps the development of the baby but also makes infant care more meaningful.

Hearing

Compared to vision the auditory system is more or less fully formed at birth. There is evidence to suggest that the fetus has been able to hear in utero for several months prior to birth (McShane, 1991). However, in general, we know less about the auditory system than the visual system and less research has been conducted on this aspect of perception.

What we do know is that infants are able to recognise their mother's voice from a very young age (see below) and are also able to discriminate quite subtle differences in language. Using a technique that involved babies sucking on a non-nutritive nipple, Eimas (1985) was able to demonstrate that babies of only a few days old could tell the difference between the sounds 'p' and 'b'. Using headphones babies were played the sound 'p' (as in puppet) when they sucked on the nipple. This continued until the infant had habituated to the sound and the sucking became less vigorous. At this point the sound was changed to 'b' (as in bag). If babies cannot hear the difference between the two sounds then you would expect no change in sucking. However, Eimas observed that the frequency of sucking went up when the sound was changed indicating that the new sound had aroused the baby's interest and the baby could tell that the two sounds were different.

Infants under one month old are also able to discriminate sounds that occur in languages other than their native tongue.

Although this ability eventually disappears, such findings have been used to suggest that human infants have an innate capacity for language learning.

Social interaction: the role of the infant

Up until now we have considered infant abilities as if they were occurring in a social vacuum. This is obviously not the case, from the moment of birth the baby enters a complex social world. She is totally dependent on others for survival and many of the capacities that babies are born with seem to indicate that they are genetically preadapted to social life. For example, we have already noted that babies see best at a distance of about eight inches, which is roughly the distance between the baby's and mother's faces while nursing. This gives the baby the best possible opportunity of gazing at his mother to engage her in social interaction and getting to know her face. This is supported by strong evidence which suggests that young infants show a visual preference for the human face.

This work was originally begun by Fantz (1961, 1963), but although his results showed that babies appeared to prefer looking at faces, they were inconclusive because of methodological difficulties. It remained unclear whether infants favoured faces or whether it was simply the complexity of the face as a visual stimulus which attracted them. The research was continued by Johnson *et al* (1991) who demonstrated that neonates only an hour old were able to track a schematic face, and showed a preference for this over a jumbled face or a blank. Johnson and Morton (1991) are cautious in their conclusions and see this ability as akin to a reflex, rather than a more complex social behaviour. It is tempting though to conclude that babies are 'hard wired' to respond to faces. But perhaps it does not really matter. The fact that babies are disposed to gaze at, and track faces helps them to engage (albeit unwittingly) in social interaction. This, like smiling and crying, enables the infant to maintain contact with the adults whose care is essential for their well being and survival.

Very young babies also seem to have the ability to discriminate between and recognise faces very quickly. As one might imagine, the mother's face seems to be very potent. Carpenter (1974) used an apparatus in which two-week-old babies were shown either their mother's face or the face of a female stranger. The infants showed a definite preference for the mother's face over the face of the stranger, demonstrating that it was not complexity alone that was attracting them. They looked longest when they were shown their mother's face plus her voice rather than her silent face and they frequently showed distress when shown the mother's face with the stranger's voice and vice versa. This study indicates that not only does the baby recognise the mother's face but also her voice. De Casper and Fifer (1980) found that infants would suck on a non-nutritive nipple in different ways in order to listen to their mother's voice reading *To think it happened on Mulberry Street* by Dr Seuss. When given the choice of hearing either a strange female voice or the voice of their mother, they consistently chose the mother, implying that the infant can discriminate between the two almost from birth.

We have seen that infants are fascinated by faces and appear to be attracted to them. Yet another capability that the infant demonstrates from birth is the ability to imitate the facial gestures of adults. Meltzoff and Moore (1977) first noted this. In a series of experiments they demonstrated babies imitating frowning, tongue protrusion and pursing of the lips as young as just a few days old (Meltzoff and Moore, 1989). Although some researchers have argued that this simply indicates a reflexive response, Meltzoff and Moore suggest that the behaviour is more complex than this, involving what they call Active Intermodal Matching or AIM. They claim that in order to imitate the facial gestures they observe in the adult model, the baby must be able to convert what it sees through the visual 'channel' into movement. The baby must also recognise the correct part of their own body to move. According to Meltzoff this implies that at some level they must recognise that they also have a mouth, tongue, eyebrows, just like the adult they are looking at. These movements of the mouth area, in particular, have led some researchers to suggest that these movements could be the precursors to language.

If we take all of these things that infants 'do', crying, smiling, tracking and watching faces, imitating facial gestures, recognising the mother's face and voice and so on, it all seems to add up to the fact that babies easily 'slot in' to a social situation. This is obviously good news in terms of survival.

So far, we have considered what the infant does and not how parents respond to the infant behaviour. Let us now consider the part that the adults play in this.

Social interaction: the role of the adult

Schaffer (1996) argues that the most urgent task for parents during the first few weeks of life is to regulate the biological processes of the infant and most social exchanges take place around this. He is very clear that parents follow the child's developmental agenda and not vice versa and are skilled in dovetailing their own behaviour to accomodate the infant's needs. For example, we have seen that babies are attracted to faces and will spend some time looking at them. When the mother observes the baby's interest she will talk and perhaps make exaggerated facial gestures in order to keep the infant's attention. Once the infant indicates that they need time out by looking away, the mother ceases her interaction and waits until once again the baby demonstrates interest.

Similar interaction patterns can be observed during feeding. Wolff (1966) noticed that when babies feed they tend to do so in bursts. Each burst of sucking is followed by a brief pause before the onset of the next burst. What Kaye (1977) found interesting was the mother's behaviour. He observed that she tended to be quite passive while the infant was in a burst phase, but when the infant paused she would become active. Sometimes this involved talking to the baby or rocking her or stroking her cheek. The mother's activity continued until sucking restarted when once again she would become still. Schaffer (1996) suggests that such sequencing of dovetailed turn taking behaviour is not dissimilar to adult conversational turn taking, where one person talks while the other listens. He proposes that such sequencing could be the embryonic form of other turn-taking activities that adults engage in. He also noted that turn-taking games continue with older infants, such as peep-po, handing objects to the infant and waiting for the baby to hand them back and so on.

Snow (1972) looked at another aspect of maternal behaviour that is directed towards the infant. She was particularly interested in the precursors of language and noted that mother's respond to infant noises and gestures as if the baby was really trying to communicate something to them. In addition, mothers build a turn taking sequence into this. For example, having spoken to the baby the mother waits for a moment until the infant makes some kind of noise or gesture. She then treats this gesture 'as if' the baby were making some meaningful comment and taking a 'turn' in a conversational exchange. The mother then 'replies' to the gesture and carries on the conversation. The following is an example of a fairly typical interaction.

Mother:	*Hello there! Are you a hungry girl?*
Baby:	Gurgles
Mother:	*Are you ready for your milk?*
Baby:	Waves arms
Mother:	*I thought so*

Once again, it appears that adults behave in a way that helps to initiate the baby into the social world from a very early age. Adult and infant are engaged in a complex sequencing of behaviours that begins at birth and accumulates over the years in both depth and complexity to become the foundations of later social interaction.

Bonding

There is some confusion among health professionals about human bonding and what it really is. The majority of midwives that I talk to believe it is a genuine phenomenon with a clear biological basis and fear about lack of bonding is frequently a cause of anxiety in mothers who for some reason have to be separated from their babies at birth. It is important to be clear that when we talk about bonding in humans we are talking about an emotional bond that the mother is presumed to make towards her infant. It is assumed that this happens in a sensitive period shortly after birth but, as we shall see, the evidence for such a mechanism existing in humans is rather weak.

There is ethological evidence from animal studies that indicates bonding occurs in a variety of species. Lorenz (1937) noted that goslings bond (or imprint) on the mother shortly after hatching. Herd animals, such as goats, horses and sheep also seem to form mother/ infant bonds shortly after birth. Obviously in these species there are good reasons why such bonding should occur, it makes sense for the mother to recognise her offspring and for the young animal to stay close to her. This has the advantage of keeping the animal safe and near the source of food, thereby maximising its chances of survival.

Klaus and Kennell (1976) noting the existence of such mechanisms in other species considered whether something similar might occur in humans and carried out a study to try to clarify this. They believed that close skin to skin contact following birth would increase the likelihood of the formation of a maternal bond, thus improving the subsequent mother/infant relationship.They compared two groups of young mothers. The control group simply had normal contact with their newborn during their stay in hospital. The experimental group, on the other hand, had an hour of skin to skin contact in the three hours after birth and a further five hours in the next three days. When the subjects were followed up a month later it was found that mothers who had extra contact with their babies showed a greater attachment to their offspring on a variety of measures and this effect appeared to persist even a year later. The control group did not show such strong attachments even though they would have had many opportunites of being close to their infants. It seemed as if the critical period for bonding was just after birth. Some years later Klaus and Kennell's findings were replicated in a Swedish study involving forty-two middle class Swedish mothers (de Chateau, 1987).

The human bonding hypothesis had a major impact on the way mothers and babies were treated in hospital. Whereas in the past babies were taken from the mother almost immediately after birth, hospital routines have now changed. Mothers are encouraged to hold their babies immediately after birth and to breast feed and cuddle them. For most mothers and babies this was a positive move enabling the mother to enjoy contact with her new baby, however, it created difficulties and anxieties for those for whom such close contact was impossible.

There were also methodological problems with the studies too. Klaus and Kennell's results could be explained simply by the Hawthorne effect. This refers to the well documented finding that people in psychological studies show changes in behaviour simply because they know that they are part of a study and are being observed. The Hawthorne effect, rather than the close contact after birth, could be the explanation for the enhanced mother/infant relationship in the experimental group. Other studies have also failed to replicate Klaus and Kennell's results (Durkin, 1995).

It is probably too simplistic to explain a mother's attachment to her baby in terms of a 'sensitive' period after birth. As we have noted previously, birth is not simply a biological process but a complex social and cultural event and the way the mother responds to her newborn child will depend on a number of factors. In addition, human relationships are not static one-way affairs, both mother and baby are engaged in a dynamic interaction that is constantly evolving and changing. Some women who are brave enough to admit it will say that they felt almost nothing but exhaustion after their baby was born and they did not feel loving towards them until some time after the birth. There is no evidence to suggest that mothers who cannot have close skin to skin contact with their babies because they are sick do not bond well with them. The existence of such a mechanism would also preclude fathers (who have not gone through the process of giving birth) and adoptive parents from bonding with their babies.

It is impossible to conclude that if a mother fails to bond with her infant at birth, this pattern will persist over time. In fact, it could be argued that bonding might be counter-productive in humans, preventing others from caring for offspring who have lost their mothers. Everything that social psychologists know about human relationships indicate that they are more flexible than this involving social and cultural influences and an individual's own thinking and reasoning processes. I must agree with Durkin who concludes that although everyone agrees that the early parent child relationship is an important one, '... the notion of a sensitive period for maternal bonding is not widely accepted' (1995 p. 91).

Can postnatal depression have a negative impact on child development ?

In the following chapter, we will consider the devastating effects of postnatal depression (PND), but largely from the perspective of the mother. Evidence is also accumulating that children of mothers who have suffered from postnatal depression may experience cognitive and emotional delays, behavioural problems and difficulty in forming a secure attachment to the mother. As we shall see, the evidence from these studies is difficult to interpret and, for reasons that I discuss later, I remain slightly sceptical about the direct influence that postnatal depression is assumed to have on infant and child development. Before I go on to talk about this, let's look at the evidence that has been put forward that suggests that PND has a detrimental affect on infant development.

The rationale for studying the impact of maternal postnatal depression on child development comes from two sources, the work that has been done on mother/infant interaction (see above) and the evidence that psychiatric problems in parents can have negative consequences for children (Rutter, 1989; Radke-Yarrow, 1990)

We have already seen how salient the human face is for infants and *Chapter 5* notes how important the face is for reflecting a wide range of emotions. For many years psychologists have been aware that infant's are sensitive to the emotional states of others, particularly the primary caretaker (Murray and Trevarthen, 1985; Tronick *et al*, 1986). In normal mother/infant interaction, babies show a relaxed posture, smile and gurgle and move arms and legs freely. The picture is quite different when mothers are asked to gaze at their baby with an expressionless face. This behaviour evokes a tense posture in the infant and virtually no smiling. Field *et al* (1988) carried out an experiment in which they asked mothers who were not suffering from postnatal depression to interact with their babies 'as if' they were depressed. These mothers were allowed to talk to their infants but in a flat voice with little or no facial expression. In this situation the researchers reported that after a short time, the infants too began to look depressed and even interacted with a non-depressed adult in a depressed way. Field *et al* (1985) also noted that babies with depressed mothers showed fewer positive facial expressions and more protest behaviour than a matched sample of non-depressed controls. Research of this kind has raised the question of whether infants who are exposed to a mother whose affect is permanently sad and quiet because she is suffering from depression, may experience long-term psychological difficulties.

Lyons-Ruth *et al* (1986) carried out a study on fifty-six women from low income families. This group was chosen for investigation because previous research had indicated that women from such a background were more likely to suffer from depression than more affluent women. Half of the women in the study had been referred because they were experiencing difficulties in relating to their offspring as well as economic and social stresses. This group was matched with a group of women from a low income community sample who were not experiencing relationship difficulties with their babies. All the women in the sample had a baby under the age of twelve months and they were studied until their children were eighteen months old.

The researchers measured a number of variables, which included assessment of maternal depression, assessment of maternal family history, maternal behaviour at home, infant development, maternal intelligence and infant attachment security. It was found that depressed mothers were more irritable and resentful of their children and less affectionate and warm, they were also more critical and demanding than the matched controls. The infants of these mothers had lower scores on mental and motor development scales when they were tested at twelve months, with differences between infants of the least depressed and most depressed mothers exceeding ten points on the scale. Infants of depressed mothers were also insecurely attached, but this was also true of infants of some mothers who were not depressed. Surprisingly, Lyons-Ruth *et al* (1986) found no relationship between the observational data on maternal behaviour and infant development, although there was a relationship between maternal IQ and infant development. Although this study demonstrates a link between maternal depression and lower development scores, it is not clear what aspect of the mother's behaviour (if any) is causing this.

Coghill *et al* (1986) studied 119 primiparous women from early pregnancy to four years postpartum. They measured the cognitive development of the ninety-nine children remaining in the study at four years old, and found that the twenty-two children of the mothers who had been depressed in the first postnatal year scored significantly lower on the McCarthy scales of cognitive development than the other children. Cognitive delay was also found to be related to parental conflict, a history of paternal psychiatric problems and low socio-economic status. In their conclusion, these authors correctly point out that causal relationships cannot be inferred from positive correlation between variables. They nevertheless go on to argue that the interdependence of postnatal depression,

> *with marital problems, father's psychiatric history, and parental social class point to ways in which maternal postnatal depression might exert its impact.*

> (Coghill *et al*, 1986, p. 1167)

In a subsequent study of the same group of mothers and children, Caplan *et al* (1989) considered whether behavioural disturbance in the children at four years of age was related to maternal postnatal depression. Their findings indicated that although there was a relationship between depression at 0–3 months postpartum, the biggest predictor of child behaviour problems was concurrent maternal depression. As in their earlier study, there was once again a relationship between behavioural disturbance in the children and marital disharmony and paternal psychiatric problems. In this paper the authors comment that, 'maternal depression may **reflect** or **cause** greater marital problems' (author's emphasis, p. 821). Having acknowledged this, and the fact that other studies point to the significance of family discord and hostility that accounts for the relationship between parental psychiatric disorder and disturbance in the child, they nevertheless go on to conclude:

The early detection and treatment of maternal depression is important, not only to relieve distress in the mothers and their spouses but also perhaps to prevent disturbance in the children.

Gotlib, Whitten *et al* (1989) studied twenty-five depressed and twenty-five non-depressed mothers and their two-month-old infants. The babies were assessed using the Bayley scales of infant development and mothers completed questionnaires on infant temperament and difficulties associated with infant care. In general, women in the depressed group had experienced fewer years of education. Depressed women did not rate their infants as more temperamentally difficult than non-depressed women but they did report more difficulties with infant care and perceived their infants as more bothersome. The babies of the depressed mothers generally achieved lower scores on the Bayley scales of infant development and responded more negatively to testing and became agitated and fretful more quickly than the infants of the non-depressed mothers.

Murray (1992) studied a much larger sample of 113 mother/infant pairs. Women were divided into four groups:

- no previous history of depression and no depression since delivery (N=42)
- no history of depression but who had experienced depression since childbirth (N=40)
- a previous history of depression but none since delivery (N=14)
- a previous history of depression and depression since delivery (N=21).

This sample was slightly skewed in favour of higher socioeconomic classes with 60% of the sample coming from social classes I, II and III (non-manual and students) and the remaining 40% coming from social classes III (manual), IV and V.

One hundred and eleven of the 113 infants were assessed at eighteen months old on a variety of scales. The findings indicated that those infants whose mothers were postnatally depressed were more insecurely attached to their mothers and performed worse on an object concept task (the ability to search for an object when it has been placed out of sight). There was only slight evidence of behaviour problems as shown by severe sleep disturbance and no relationship was found between postnatal depression and general cognitive and language development.

Given our assumptions about the centrality of the mother/infant relationship in child development, it appears logical to assume that if a mother is withdrawn and depressed then the infant will be affected in some negative way. However, perhaps we are being too hasty in assuming that it is the existence of postnatal depression in the mother *per se* that is having a direct negative impact on the development of the infant. This point may be seen more clearly if we begin to analyse some of the details of the studies that have just been described.

Almost all the studies that have been discussed have used relatively small sample sizes. Frequently, fewer than thirty depressed women and their children have been included in the studies. This is understandable because depressed women may be reluctant to participate in such studies, and when a sample of women are studied longitudinally it is impossible to predict how many of them will become depressed. However, findings from such small samples cannot easily be extrapolated to the wider population. Moreover, some studies have used atypical populations deliberately choosing low income samples because women from this section of society are known to be at greater risk of depression. These women are also likely to experience more economic and social stresses and to be less well educated, a factor that is known to relate to child development. When a larger scale study that samples a more representative group is undertaken, such as the one by Murray (1992), it is more difficult to demonstrate the relationship between postnatal depression and deficits in child development.

This highlights the difficulty in teasing out what exactly is causing the problem (if any) in the children. Despite the fact that all researchers acknowledge that the existence of a positive correlation between two measures cannot be taken to infer causality, they persist in assuming that PND and child development are causally related in some way. To take an example, the studies by Coghill *et al* (1986) and Caplan *et al* (1989) both noted the existence of a relationship between psychiatric problems in the father and cognitive delays in the children. These authors, however, still persisted with their conclusion that it was the depression in the mother that was the significant factor in the cognitive delays observed in the children. In reality, these authors are in no position to draw such a conclusion, as they have only demonstrated a relationship between postnatal depression and aspects of child development. It is equally possible that it is as much the father's psychiatric condition as the mother's depression that is having an effect on the children. More realistically, it is probably a complex interaction between all of these variables.

Certainly a mother with postnatal depression will put an emotional strain on the whole family. Meighan *et al* (1999) looked at father's experiences and found that their inability to fix the problem led to anger and frustration. The fathers in this study also felt confused and fearful and found it difficult to understand the change that had taken place in their partner.

Murray and Cooper (1996a) argue that there are several possible explanations for why there could be a link between postnatal depression and child development. Firstly, there might be a direct influence from exposure to the symptoms of depression in the mother. Secondly, the effect could come from the mother's inability to respond positively to her infant because of her depression; and thirdly, there could be environmental factors which are causing the mother's depression and are indirectly having an impact on the infant. Finally, there could be genetic or constitutional factors at play. There are studies that have shown all of these possible explanations to be influential but few, if any, of the studies that have been considered have taken all of these factors into account.

In a more recent paper Murray *et al* (1996b) comment:

> *It may be premature to conclude, on the basis of the work published to date, that postnatal depression generally poses a risk for the longer term cognitive development of the child.*

(p. 927)

They conclude from a follow-up study of ninety-five mother/infant pairs that when the children were tested at five years of age there was no evidence of an adverse effect of postnatal depression. This was true even among sub-groups of children previously thought to be vulnerable, such as boys and children from low SES families. A meta-analysis of nine studies was carried out by Beck (1998). This was aimed at determining the magnitude of the effect of postpartum depression on the emotional development of children under the age of twelve months. The conclusion of this analysis was that postpartum depression had a small but significant effect on children's cognitive and emotional development.

There is also some evidence to suggest that postnatal depression affects children's social-emotional adjustment to school. Sinclair and Murray (1998) found that postnatal and recent depression was linked with raised level of disturbance in school, particularly boys and Wright *et al* (1999) found that maternal depression is related to behaviour problems at school

Rather than looking at the relationship between PND and child development some studies have attempted to consider the mechanisms by which such an effect could operate, that is, if there is a relationship between PND and child development, what aspects of the mother's behaviour are significant? It would seem that the most likely explanation is the lack of stimulation that the infant receives. The mother who is depressed finds it difficult to respond in a lively and positive way to her infant. She tends to speak less frequently and her facial expressions are flat and more impassive than if she were feeling well. It is this lack of stimulation that appears to affect babies the most when their mothers become depressed. It would also appear that there is a sex difference in the way boys and girls react to their mother's depression. Murray *et al* (1999) and Wright *et al* (2000) have reported similar findings. Carter *et al* (2001) found that maternal depressive symptoms were associated with problem behaviours and lower competencies in boys but it was the quality of the mother/infant interaction that seemed to influence girls.

By now you might be forgiven for feeling rather confused about the issue of postnatal depression and child development. What is the answer: does it or does it not lead to difficulties in development? Despite, or perhaps, because of the complexity of the findings in the studies that have been described it is possible to reach a conclusion, although it may not be as neat as some people might wish. It seems to me unlikely that postnatal depression alone leads to negative outcomes for any individual child. After all, an infant is rarely alone with the mother for twenty-four hours a day, seven days a week and it is likely that other people with whom the baby will interact will provide sufficient social stimulation for normal development to occur. When postnatal depression is combined with other negative life events, such as; economic and social stress, psychiatric illness in the father, marital difficulties, birth complications, negative temperament in the infant etc. this could lead to problems. In such cases, postnatal depression in the mother if it is profound and long-term may be the most significant factor, but one would still need to consider whether other negative aspects of the woman's situation were actually contributing to her depressed state.

This has necessarily been only a brief description of the literature on the relationship between postnatal depression and child development. A full account of many of the earlier studies on this subject can be found in Murray and Cooper (1997).

Conclusion

In this chapter I have briefly reviewed our current state of knowledge about the abilities of the newborn. We know quite a lot about infant perception and we believe that the baby comes into the world with predispositions to perceive the world in certain ways and to interact with those who will care for them. As a midwife, you have only brief contact with the newborn child and her mother but I think that during this time a significant contribution can be made to the mother/infant relationship.

Caring for a tiny baby is hard work and may be seen by the mother as one-sided and unrewarding. Most human relationships are reciprocal but a new baby does not seem to do very much apart from demanding a great deal of attention. When mothers are physically exhausted from the birth, they may feel unable to meet the demands of their new baby, particularly if they do not appear to get much back in return except dirty nappies and hours of crying.

This is where educating mothers about the abilities of the newborn can be helpful and midwives are in an excellent position to pass on this information. If mothers knew that right from birth the baby knows and recognises her voice, can see her face clearly when she is feeding him, and will soon be able to recognise her face and prefer to look at it rather than others, this could help her to feel that the relationship was not all one-sided. Mothers and fathers could also be shown how their babies copy facial and hand gestures, and this could encourage playful interactions, which might ease the responsibility of constant caring and also encourage the building of a positive relationship with the infant.

Although quite a lot of investment is now being put into parenting programmes such as Sure Start, to my knowledge these ideas have never been tested out in an experimental situation. It seems that if parents can be encouraged to become interested and engaged with their babies early on, then this could be helpful in easing the early days of life for both mother and baby and, in addition, might have long-term benefits.

References

Beck CT (1998) The effects of postpartum depression on child development: a meta-analysis. *Arch Psychiatric Nurs* **12**(1): 12–20

Bee H (1992) *The Developing Child.* 6th edn. Harper Collins, New York

Bremner JG (1994) *Infancy.* 2nd edn. Blackwell, Oxford

Caplan HL, Coghill SR, Alexandra H, Robson KM, Katz R, Kumar R (1989) Maternal depression and the emotional development of the child. *Br J Psychiatry* **154**: 818–22

Carpenter GC (1974) Mother's face and the newborn. *New Scientist* **61**: 742–4

Carter AS, Garrity-Roukous FE, Chazan-Cohen R, Little C, Briggs-Gowan MJ (2001) Maternal depression and comorbidity: Predicting early parenting, attachment security and toddler social-emotional problems and competencies. *J Am Acad Child Adolesc Psychiatry* **40**(1): 18–26

de Chateau P (1987) Parent-infant socialization in several Western European countries. In: Osofsky JD, ed. *Handbook of Infant Development.* Wiley, New York

Coghill KR, Caplan HL, Alexandra H, Robson KM, Kumar R (1986) Impact of maternal postnatal depression on cognitive development of young children. *Br Med J* **292**: 1165–7

De Casper AJ, Fifer WP (1980) Of human bonding: Newborns prefer their mothers' voices. *Science* **208**: 1174–6

Durkin K (1995) *Developmental Social Psychology: From infancy to old age.* Blackwell, Oxford

Eaton WO, Saudino KJ (1992) Prenatal activity as a temperament dimension? Individual differences and developmental functions in fetal movement. *Infant Behaviour Development* **15**: 57–70

Fantz RL (1961) The origins of form perception. *Sci Am* **204**(5): 66–72

Field TM, Sandberg D, Garcia R, Vega-Lair N, Goldstein S, Guy L (1985) Pregnancy problems, postpartum depression and early mother-infant interactions. *Dev Psychol* **21**: 1560–79

Field T, Healy B, Goldstein S *et al* (1988) Infants of depressed mothers show 'depressed' behaviour even with non depressed adults. *Child Dev* **59**: 1569–97

Flavell JH (1963) *The Developmental Psychology of Jean Piaget.* D Van Nostrand, New York

Fox NA, Henderson HA (1999) Does infancy matter? Predicting social behavior from infant temperament. *Infant Behaviour Development* **22**(4): 445–55

Gimas PD (1985) The perception of speech in early infancy. *Scientific American* **204**: 66–72

Gotlib IH, Whitten VE, Mount JH, Milne K, Cordy NI (1989) Prevalence rates and demographic characteristics associated with depression in pregnancy and the postpartum. *J Consul Clin Psychol* **57**(2): 269–74

Izard CE, Lawler TB, Haynes OM, Simons RG, Porges SW (1999–2000) Emotionality in early infancy predicts temperament through the second year of life. *Imagination, Cognition and Personality* **19**(3): 213–27

Johnson MH, Dziurawiec S, Ellis H, Morton J (1991) The tracking of face-like stimuli by newborn infants and its subsequent decline. *Cognition* **40**: 1–21

Johnson MH, Morton J (1991) *Biology and Cognitive Development: The case of face recognition.* Blackwell, Oxford

Kaye K (1977) Towards the origin of dialogue. In: Schaffer HR, ed. *Studies in Mother-infant Interaction.* Academic Press, London

Klaus MH, Kennell JH (1976) *Parent-infant Bonding*. Plume, New York

Lorenz KZ (1937) The companion in the bird's world. In: Sluckin W, ed. *Imprinting and Early Learning*. Methuen, London

Lyons-Ruth K, Zoll D, Connell D, Grunebaum HU (1986) The depressed mother and her one-year-old infant: Environment, interaction, attachment and infant development. In: Tronick EZ, Field T, eds. *New Directions for Child Development: Maternal depression and infant disturbance*. Jossey Bass, San Francisco: 61–82

McShane J (1991) *Cognitive Development: An information-processing approach*. Blackwell, Oxford

Meighan M, Davis M, Thomas SP, Droppleman PG (1999) Living with postpartum depression: The father's experience. *Am J Maternal/Child Nurs* **24**(4): 202–8

Meltzoff AN, Moore MK (1977) Imitation of facial and manual gestures by human neonates. *Science* **198**: 75–8

Meltzoff AN, Moore MK (1989) Imitation in newborn infants: Exploring the range of gestures imitated and the underlying mechanisms. *Dev Psychol* **25**: 954–62.

Murray L (1992) The impact of postnatal depression on infant development. *J Child Psychol Psychiatry* **33**(3): 543–61

Murray L, Trevarthen C (1985) Emotional regulation of interactions between two-month-olds and their mothers. In: Field T, Fox N, eds. *Social Perception in Infancy*. Ablex, New Jersey: 177–97

Murray L, Cooper PJ (1996a) The impact of postpartum depression on child development. *Int Rev Psychiatry* **8**: 55–63

Murray L, Hipwell R, Hooper R, Stein A., Cooper P (1996b) The cognitive development of 5-year-old children of postnatally depressed mothers. *J Child Psychol Psychiatry* **37**(8): 927–35

Murray L, Cooper PJ (1997) *Postpartum Depression and Child Development*. Guilford Press, New York

Murray L, Sinclair D, Cooper P, Ducournau P, Turner P (1999) The socioemotional development of 5-year-old children of postnatally depressed mothers. *J Child Psychol Psychiatry* **40**(8): 1259–71

Radke-Yarrow M (1990) Family environments of depressed and well parents and their children: Issues of research methods. In: Patterson GR, ed. *Depression and Aggression in Family Interaction*. Lawrence Erlbaum Associates, Hillsdale, New Jersey: 169–83

Rutter M (1989) Psychiatric disorder in parents as a risk factor for children. In: Schaffer D, Phillips I, Enger NB, eds. *Prevention of mental disorder alcohol and other drug use in children and adolescents*. Office for Substance Abuse, USDHHS, Rockville Maryland

Schaffer HR (1996) *Social Development*. Blackwell, Oxford

Sinclair D, Murray L (1998) Effects of postnatal depression on children's adjustment in school. *Br J Psychiatry* **172**: 58–63

Slater AM, Morison V (1985) Shape constancy and slant perception at birth. *Perception* **14**: 337–44

Snow CE (1972) Mother's speech to children learning language. *Child Development* **43**: 549–65

Stratton P (1982) Newborn Individuality. In: Stratton P, ed. *Psychobiology of the Human Newborn*. Wiley, Chichester

Thomas A, Chess S (1977) *Temperament and Development*. Brunner/Mazel, New York

Trevarthen C (1982) The primary motives for cooperative understanding. In: Butterworth G, Light P, eds. *Social Cognition: studies of the development of understanding*. University of Chicago Press, Chicargo

Tronick EZ, Cohn J, Shea E (1986) The transfer of affect between mothers and infants. In: Brazelton TB, Yogman MW, eds. *Affective Development in Infancy*. Ablex, New Jersey: 11–25

Wolff P (1966) The causes controls and organization of behaviour in the neonate. *Psychol Issues* 5 (Monograph No.17)

Wolff P (1969) The natural history of crying and other vocalizations in early infancy. In: Foss BM, ed. *Determinants of Infant Behaviour*. Vol 4. Methuen, London

Wright CA, George TP, Burke R, Gelfand DM, Teti DM (2000) Early maternal depression and children's adjustment to school. *Child Study Journal* 30(3): 153–68

9

Postnatal depression: exploding the Madonna myth

Depression and the maternal role

Depression at any time of life is debilitating, but it may be seen as particularly distressing when it occurs around the time of childbirth. Every year a significant number of women are affected by such negative emotional reactions after giving birth, causing anguish both to themselves and their families. It is important for health professionals to understand as much as possible about depression in pregnancy and the postpartum so that constructive help can be offered to sufferers.

Postnatal depression has been the subject of a great deal of research over the last twenty or thirty years and academics from many different disciplines, including medicine, sociology and psychology have attempted to explain what causes it (see Albright, 1993 for a review). Although much has been written about depression, there is confusion as to what postnatal depression actually is (Gotlib *et al*, 1989). It varies enormously in intensity, ranging from mild to severe, and despite all the studies that have been carried out there is still no clear understanding of the aetiology of the condition and little consensus about the symptoms, onset and prevalence.

Depression and motherhood; somehow the two things just do not seem to go together. Stereotypes of motherhood, which are culturally embedded and which subtly influence us all, conjure up visions of the serene woman, gently and devotedly caring for her child. For this woman nothing is too much trouble, nothing frustrates her or makes her feel angry. She cares selflessly for her infant who basks contentedly in its mother's love. The mother herself is happy in the knowledge that she has fulfilled the maternal role for which she has been biologically destined since girlhood. Several psycho-analytically-oriented writers have suggested why this view of motherhood is so pervasive in our culture.

Such rosy tinted images of pregnancy and motherhood can be seen everywhere, the myth that motherhood is both easy and natural pervades society (Jebali, 1993). Although we are bombarded with images of violence and hatred on television and in the newspapers as well as in art and film, we rarely see pictures of mothers who are angry or frustrated with their children; only placid women smiling beatifically upon their offspring. When we hear of mothers who have harmed their children or abandoned them we are horrified that such behaviour could have occurred (Jackson, 1994). Artists in the Western world have depicted this image of the mother as Madonna for centuries. For modern examples, go into any supermarket or newsagent where you will find many magazines devoted to 'parenting'; pick up any one of them and look at the advertisements and I can almost guarantee you will find only pictures of beautiful, clean, well dressed, happy babies being cared for by young, attractive women in affluent looking homes. The 'mothers' in the adverts look contented and pleased with their role, they certainly do not look exhausted or at their wits end. But, as any one who has had to care for very young children knows, such images are very different from the reality of motherhood and give absolutely no indication of the difficulties, nor of the negative feelings many women experience during this time of their lives.

Perhaps because of the strength of this 'maternity-as-bliss' stereotype, most midwives and health professionals, as well as women themselves, regard depression in the early stages of motherhood as an abnormal reaction to the birth of a baby; after all, becoming a mother should be the pinnacle of a woman's career. It is the role that nature intended her for. The influence of such a stereotype may even prevent women from admitting that they feel negative about themselves and their baby, leading them to suffer in silence. This chapter reviews some of the research that has considered PND as an abnormal response to motherhood and suggests an alternative explanation that is grounded in feminist theory. I will argue that negative emotions experienced during pregnancy and after childbirth can just as easily be seen as a rational response to the changes and adaptations that women have to make when they become mothers. I also suggest that midwives could play a significant role in influencing attitudes to PND and helping women understand the reasons why they become depressed.

Postnatal depression and the medical model

It is important to say a brief word about this, as it is useful to rehearse some of the assumptions made by this model before we move on. As we saw in the introductory chapter, the medical model of health and illness assumes that for every disease affecting the body and mind, there is some underlying physical cause. At any one point in time, we may not know the biological antecedent of an illness, but if we gain enough knowledge about the condition, eventually we will discover its origin. Once we have uncovered this underlying cause then we will be able to control and treat the illness by correcting the biological malfunction.

All medical conditions are studied using the assumptions of the medical model as a guide and are described in terms of their symptoms, aetiology, diagnosis, prognosis, and so on. Doctors and patients alike are anxious to predict and understand every aspect of a physical illness, so that appropriate treatment can be given and a cure effected. In general, physical illnesses are much easier to understand and describe in this way than mental conditions. For example, if we consider something like chicken pox, the picture is reasonably clear. We know that it is caused by the herpes simplex virus, we know the incubation period is about two weeks and that the symptoms will include fever and red itchy spots. We know roughly how long the patient will be ill and when they will cease to infect others. In short, we understand the biology of this illness. Sadly, it has never been so straightforward to apply the medical model to any disease affecting the human mind. Efforts to describe mental illnesses in the same way as physical illnesses have by and large failed. For example, we still do not know for sure what causes depression or schizophrenia, even though there have been numerous theories put forward ranging from genetic explanations to environmental ones.

Postnatal depression in all its forms has been similarly difficult to describe and academics differ widely about what they believe causes it. To date, there has been no theory put forward that adequately explains all the facts. The list of symptoms that has been suggested is so enormous that it ceases to be meaningful; the onset of the disease can be any time during the first year after the birth of the baby. Although we have ideas about risk factors, we still have no way of accurately predicting who is likely to suffer from postnatal depression, puerperal psychosis or the blues.

The variety of emotional reactions that follow birth

Giving birth seems to have the capacity to precipitate extreme emotional reactions in some women and parturition has been shown to be a 'risk factor' for psychiatric illness.

> ... *childbirth has the highest relative risk of any factor so far measured in psychiatry.*

(Brockington, 1996, p. 222)

Negative emotional reactions following childbirth have been divided into three categories (Chalmers and Chalmers, 1986; Harding, 1989). This is not totally clearcut as there is some argument about whether these are three distinct 'conditions' or simply a continuum of psychological distress ranging from mild to severe (Hannah *et al*, 1992). For the moment, it is clearer to maintain the distinction and describe the three types of postpartum mental disturbances as if they were separate and distinct clinical entities.

Puerperal or postpartum psychosis

This is the most severe of the three conditions and is fortunately, relatively uncommon. It affects about one or two women per 1000 and this rate appears to be consistent across time and between cultures (Kumar, 1994). It is generally assumed that it is caused by some biological factor, although this remains elusive (Appleby *et al*, 1996). Symptoms are dramatic and women can experience the whole range of psychotic behaviours including, delusions, hallucinations, mania, catatonia and severe depression. Symptoms are so severe that urgent psychiatric treatment is usually required.

> ... *almost every psychotic symptom is found in these (postnatal) psychoses. The delusions cover the whole gamut of morbid ideas, although some are especially related to the theme of childbirth, eg. megalomaniac ideas about the identity of the baby, or persecutory ideas involving changelings. Some of the less common delusions have also been observed, eg. delusional misidentification. Verbal hallucinations, thought insertion, echo phenomena, thought broadcasting and 'made' impulses occur, often accompanied by ideas of control or possession. Catatonic features, ie.*

imperviousness to the environment and catalepsy have been
emphasised as particularly common.

(Brockington, 1996, p. 209)

The onset is usually within two weeks of giving birth, but can be up to three months postpartum. Some have argued that there is a lucid period of two days after parturition, but not everyone agrees, as onset can be immediately after the birth, at weaning, and at the time of the first period, in fact, at almost any time in the postnatal period. Women are extremely ill. They usually require hospitalisation and may be of some danger to themselves and to their babies. They may be very depressed and suicide attempts are not uncommon. Appleby *et al* (1998) showed that severe postpartum psychiatric disorder is associated with a high rate of deaths from both natural and unnatural causes, particularly suicide. The team noted that the risk is especially high in the first postnatal year, when the suicide risk is increased seventy-fold. This kind of postnatal illness is not difficult to diagnose, everyone around the woman who is suffering knows that there is something seriously wrong with her, she is not herself and is not behaving normally.

The prognosis is good; nearly all women recover from it, some within a few days, others in a few months. Pfuhlmann *et al* (1999) examined thirty-nine women who had suffered from a severe first-episode psychiatric illness six to twenty-six years later. Although relapse was common, following another pregnancy or delivery, only four patients had never fully recovered.

As with the other postnatal mental illnesses that will be discussed later in this chapter, there is uncertainty about the cause, although a biological explanation of some kind is usually favoured. As with the less severe postnatal depression, the biological mechanisms remain unclear. Hormonal changes have inevitably been implicated, oestrogen, progesterone, and cortisol have all been suggested as likely precipitators, but there is no clear relationship between changing levels of these and the incidence of puerperal psychosis. As Appleby *et al* (1996) comment:

... it is widely believed that the massive hormonal changes
following childbirth trigger affective disorder in women
who are genetically vulnerable to such illness. The precise
mechanism remains unknown...

(p. 927)

Evidence has been gathered that suggests that there is some hereditary tendency as mental illness is more common in the families of those who suffer from puerperal psychosis. At this moment in time there is still no clear biological explanation. Although clinical trials are scarce, patients have been treated with electro-convulsive therapy (ECT), lithium, sedatives, hormones, counselling and psychotherapy.

The 'Blues'

These are less severe and very common. It has been suggested that as many as 80% of women experience a period of emotional lability a few days after giving birth (Oakley and Chamberlain, 1981), although other authors argue a more modest 60% (Harris, 1994; 1996). Women are described as being emotional and irrational, often bursting into tears for no apparent reason. Because the blues occurs at a predictable time after parturition, there is more evidence for a biological explanation but, despite a great deal of research, there is still no known cause.

Although the blues has been specifically linked with birth, there is evidence to suggest that a similar period of emotional lability occurs in other groups who have experienced a traumatic event. Levy (1994) compared a group of male and female postoperative patients with women who had recently given birth. She found that a similar period of dysphoria occurred in postoperative women and to a lesser extent to postoperative men, indicating that the blues is not unique to postpartum women, but could be a normal response to a stressful event. There were some differences in onset with the maternity blues occurring three to four days after birth, while postoperative blues tended to occur immediately after the operation and then diminish.

However, the symptoms were similar in the two groups including; depression, tension, anxiety, lack of concentration, restlessness, confusion, tiredness, irritability, anorexia, forgetfulness, insomnia, headache and dreaming.

What is interesting about this study is that most clinicians and nurses must be aware of emotional reactions in postoperative patients and this is accepted as an understandable response to the stress of surgery and a normal part of recovery. There is no attempt to explain it in terms of hormonal changes or other biological mechanisms. This begs the question; why is the blues regarded as unusual in women who have given birth, but acceptable in postoperative patients? I will leave you to think about this for the moment, but will return to it later in the chapter.

Postnatal depression or postpartum depression is less severe than puerperal psychosis but it is also more common and affects a greater number of women. Oakley (1979) subdivides it into:

a. Depression which occurs when the mother arrives home with the baby, often accompanied by anxiety lasting a week or two.
b. Depressed affect that comes and goes. Women have good and bad times and this occurs around three months postpartum.
c. A more severe clinical depression that affects the woman more deeply and is accompanied by other symptoms common in depression, such as loss of weight, sleep disturbance etc.

Although there is some argument in the literature about whether this depression in the postpartum is different from depression occurring at any other time of life (Glover, 1992), this 'type' of emotional upheaval following birth has been even more difficult to define than puerperal psychosis and has received the greatest amount of attention in the research literature.

What is postnatal depression (PND)?

At face value this seems a simple enough question which should have a reasonably straightforward answer. I ought to be able to trot out a definition at this point: Postnatal depression is... but unfortunately, it is not as easy as this. Although most people in the street could tell you what they *think* PND is and might even be able to suggest underlying causes and symptoms, a medically precise definition remains elusive (Gotlib *et al*, 1989).

> *Despite all that has been written on this topic* (PND), *however considerable confusion remains about the definition and indeed the existence of postpartum depression as a unique disorder.*

> (Gotlib *et al*, 1989, p. 269)

In his book *Motherhood and Mental Illness* Brockington (1996) comments that:

> *One must examine, with scepticism, the scientific value of* ***postnatal depression****.*

> (p. 170, author's emphasis)

and,

> *The concept of 'postnatal depression' does not emerge*
> *from thirty years of research with much scientific credit.*

(p. 173)

At first these statements seem rather shocking, after all, we do know what PND is, don't we? But Brockington's remarks reflect the fact that, although nobody doubts the existence of mental distress following childbirth, we still do not have an understanding of the aetiology of the condition, nor of the symptoms and causes. We remain unclear about whether PND is qualitatively different from depression occurring at any other time of life, whether it is biologically caused (Glover, 1992) or induced by psychosocial risk factors and what precisely the symptoms are.

Brockington goes on to argue that the term itself could be dangerous in that it leads us to assume that there is a specific condition that can be identified and treated in a reasonably straight-forward way and yet, to date, we have no sure-fire way of recognising or treating women who are suffering from PND. How can we, when we still do not fully understand the symptoms or what causes it?

Symptoms of postnatal depression

A wide variety of symptoms have been suggested as being indicative of postnatal depression. These include:

- tiredness
- weepiness
- over-sensitivity
- feelings of helplessness or hopelessness
- excessive dependency
- feelings of inadequacy, anxiety and despair
- compulsive thoughts
- feelings of a 'change' in oneself
- feelings that 'life will never be the same again'
- a lack of drive and energy
- loss of interest in sexual activities
- irrational fears about the baby's safety or the mother's health.

The list is so long that its usefulness as a diagnostic tool is questionable (Chalmers and Chalmers, 1986). In addition, nearly all the symptoms which are assumed to be symptomatic of underlying mental disorder could, if looked at in a different way, be considered as a normal response to the demands of motherhood.

For example, tiredness is understandable given the lack of sleep most mothers of young children have, weepiness is a normal response to an emotionally exhausting experience and over-sensitivity and feelings of helplessness and hopelessness are acceptable responses to the demands of coping with a completely new situation for which you are not prepared. Childbirth itself is exhausting (that is why it is called labour) and women get very little chance to recover from it before they return to their homes where they may be expected to carry on as normal. If they have had a Caesarean section then tiredness may be even worse. There is no other abdominal operation where you would be required to return to normal activity as quickly. In general, you are instructed to rest, take several months off work and not lift heavy objects. Although the newly delivered mother may try to do all of these things, in reality, unless you have a lot of help, it is impossible. Looking after a small baby is physically exhausting too, a woman may find that she has very little time to sit down and rest. Is it any wonder that she feels tired? There is really nothing unusual about it, anyone in the same position would feel similarly exhausted.

Women are not well prepared for the impact that motherhood will have on their lives and become distressed when they find that being a mother leaves them worn out and depressed. The majority of women believe that they should be able to cope and feel inadequate when they find that they cannot. Feeling that 'life will never be the same again' is an accurate reflection of reality. Life for the new mother has changed completely and will not be the same as it was before the baby was born. For many women this will be a cause for joy, but it may bring negative feelings for others. Women do have to give up many activities that they enjoyed before the baby came along and adapt to numerous changes. Although it is now common for women to return to work after having children, many give up their jobs because of lack of adequate childcare. Even if women do return to work it is not straightforward, women worry about the childcare arrangements that they have made and often feel guilty about leaving the baby in the care of another. Leaving work or working part-time could mean that family finances become restricted making it difficult to do things that were previously taken for granted.

Loss of libido and difficulty in sleeping are also understandable. If you are sore and uncomfortable from stitches or a difficult labour, then you will not relish the idea of sex and sleep may be difficult if you are constantly listening to hear if your baby is about to wake up. Many women have to cope with babies who sleep little and cry a lot. Armstrong *et al* (1998) found that in women who experienced postnatal depression when their infants were slightly older, there was a link between their depressed mood and sleep deprivation. Once children were sleeping better, symptoms of postnatal depression improved. In addition to lack of sleep, women may have other small children to look after and have to manage this, often with minimal support from other people. Despite the advent of the 'new man' the burden of caring for a new baby still falls mainly on the woman. There is no break from motherhood and even if a woman is ill herself, she has to carry on caring for her baby and coping with its demands. In fact, if one considers the adjustments that women have to make to cope with motherhood a period of feeling 'depressed' is understandable, so why is it regarded as unusual?

I have just taken a few examples here, but you can go through the whole list and treat it in the same vein. Once you begin to see the symptoms of PND in this light some of them become absurd to the point of being laughable. 'Feelings of a change in oneself'? Of course there has been a change, you have become a mother and changed your status forever. 'Feeling that life will never be the same again'? Too right, it will never be the same again, you will always now feel responsible for this life that you have produced. This does not reflect abnormal thinking, it is true that life will never be the same again and this may only hit home once a woman is experiencing what life is really like with a small baby.

In summary, any of the symptoms described above, may be caused by biological upheaval, but could equally well be related to the considerable adjustments most women have to make when they become mothers. As symptoms that could be used to diagnose postnatal depression they are not terribly helpful. Not only is the list too long to be meaningful, but in addition many symptoms are not in fact abnormal or irrational but reflect a woman coming to terms with a major life change. As Nicolson (1990) states:

> ... *childbirth and early motherhood typically demand physical and psychological adjustment, which is a normal consequence of these experiences.*

> (p. 693)

The symptoms outlined above can only be seen as abnormal when they are viewed in the context of the discourse that mothering is normal and natural and that women should take to it like ducks to water. Jane Ussher, who has written about PND at some length makes a comment that has always stuck in my mind because it so clearly highlights our unrealistic expectations of women's adjustment to motherhood. She argues that if we encountered someone (male or female) who was looking after an elderly relative who needed twenty-four-hour care, was incontinent, had to be fed, was irascible and bad tempered and needed attention throughout the night, we would not be at all surprised if this individual was also suffering from depression. In fact, we would probably be surprised if they were not depressed (Ussher, 1992b). Yet, health professionals continue to believe that depression following childbirth is an abnormal response to motherhood.

Prevalence of postnatal depression

There is a wide variation in both the reported prevalence and onset of postnatal depression. While all studies agree that it occurs commonly, estimates of prevalence vary enormously. *Table 9.1* shows a comparison of results from several different studies that have been carried out over the last few decades.

Table 9.1: Comparison of studies of postnatal depression

Author	Prevalence	Time after delivery
Pitt, 1968	10.8%	Six weeks
Paykel *et al*, 1980	20%	Six weeks
Cox *et al*, 1982	13%	Three to five months
O'Hara *et al*, 1984	12%	Two months
Kumar and Robson, 1984	17%	Three months
Watson *et al*, 1984	16%	Six weeks
Cooper *et al*, 1988	8.8%	Six months
Gotlib *et al*, 1989	24.8%	Ten days

The variation in reported prevalence reflects two methodological problems, both stemming from the lack of an adequate definition of postnatal depression. Firstly, lack of a precise definition makes it hard to identify accurately women who are suffering from PND and secondly, studies have used different diagnostic criteria to demonstrate the existence of postnatal depression in the women who have participated in them. This lack of a firm definition and the wide range of symptoms means that it is almost impossible for health professionals to agree about whether a woman is postnatally depressed or not. The result of this is that precise estimates of the prevalence of depression following childbirth remain difficult to pinpoint and it may be more common than many studies suggest. When self-report measures have been used they have generally yielded higher prevalence rates. McIntosh (1993) found that when depression was defined as depressed mood for at least two weeks at some stage during the first nine months postpartum, 63% of the women in his sample reported experiencing depression and Catalbiano and Catalbiano (1996) found that 42.4% of mothers in their sample reported that they had experienced some postnatal depression. If, as these studies suggest, about 50% of women experience depression in the early stages of motherhood, then this finding supports the idea that it may be seen as part of the adaptation a woman has to make to becoming a new mother.

There is another issue that makes it difficult to be accurate about prevalence rates. We see in the studies of McIntosh and Catalbiano and Catalbiano that when women self-report, prevalence rates appear higher but there is another difference in these studies, both used retrospective self-reports of postnatal depression. Although in general, retrospective reports can be criticised because they lack accuracy (people's memories are notoriously bad), it is possible that prevalence rates appear higher in such retrospective studies, for a different reason. Many women are reluctant to admit being post-natally depressed and will actively try to disguise it. There are at least two reasons for this. Firstly, women are afraid that the baby will be taken away from them. Sometimes when women are feeling depressed they may wish that the baby will not wake up or will simply disappear. It is extremely unlikely that the mother will actually harm the baby, but she fears that if she admits these feelings and something then happens that she will be held responsible. Secondly, women feel guilty about being depressed. They feel that they are lucky to have a beautiful and healthy baby and that they should be enjoying motherhood. Many women feel that there is no one they can turn to who will understand what they are going through.

Another difficulty with comparing studies of PND is that different scales have been used to measure it, many of which were not specifically designed for postpartum depression, but were for identifying depression at other times of life. Well known scales such as the Social Anxiety and Depression Scale (SADS) (Bedford and Foulds, 1978), the General Health Questionnaire (Goldberg *et al*,

1970; Goldberg, 1972) and the Beck Depression Inventory (Beck *et al*, 1961) have all been used, but questions on these scales were often inappropriate and not specific enough for the particular difficulties women face in the postpartum period. Also, many of the physiological changes associated with depression (such as sleep disturbance) might be considered normal after birth (Cox *et al*, 1987). It has also been suggested that the results obtained from these scales were not reliable, as they had been standardised on an inappropriate sample (people with general depression, rather than postnatal depression). Since 1987 the Edinburgh Postnatal Depression Scale (EPDS) (Cox *et al*, *ibid*) has been used in most studies to demonstrate the existence of depression in women after birth. This is a brief questionnaire, which is easy to administer and has been found to be successful in screening women for postnatal depression and so one might hope to see greater consistency between studies in the future. The only disadvantage about the EPDS is that the questions are quite transparent, it would be easy for a woman to disguise the fact that she was depressed, if she did not want to admit it and this might make prevalence rates appear lower than they actually are.

Onset of postnatal depression

The onset of PND is variable and as *Table 9.1* shows it has been measured at different times in the postnatal period. Some studies assume that postnatal depression proper must begin in the first six weeks after birth while other authors argue that it can occur at any time during the first postnatal year. Chalmers and Chalmers (1986) suggest that this apparent variation in onset argues against PND having a biological cause.

> *All women giving birth undergo hormonal changes, but only a few become depressed. If hormones were the sole cause of depression, then one would expect the relation-ship to be somewhat more distinct.*
>
> (Chalmers and Chalmers, 1986, p. 96)

If, for example, it was due to some variation in hormones it should always occur within a similar time frame. This has led certain researchers to suggest that postnatal depression that occurs in the first few weeks postpartum is different in some way from postnatal depression that occurs some months after birth. But this seems to be straining theory to fit observation, rather than theory predicting what is observed.

If we regard PND as a response to the demands of motherhood, then it is quite understandable that it could occur at different times postnatally, onset would depend not so much on the time after birth but on an individual woman's situation and experience of motherhood. For some women depression may occur in the immediate post birth period, while for others it may not happen until her baby is older.

What is the cause of PND?

Researchers have justified searching for the causes of PND in terms of identifying women who are at 'risk' so that they can be singled out and treated more quickly and efficiently. We have seen that the symptoms of PND are many and diverse, presenting a confused picture of what it really is. In addition, it has been difficult to be accurate about the prevalence and onset of the disorder. In view of this, it is hardly surprising that the causes of postnatal depression have also proved difficult to identify. Explanations range from the purely biological where women are seen as being the victims of their hormones, to psychosocial and feminist explanations.

Those coming from a medical orientation believe that there is an underlying biological cause of postnatal depression and over the years several hormones, biochemical factors and also thyroid deficiency have been implicated, but to date there have been no consistent findings. Despite this, the search for a simple, biological explanation goes on.

The rationale for a biological explanation seems logical enough. Following birth, there is a major change in hormone levels and this, it is assumed, creates the mental distress. Both oestrogen and progesterone have been suggested as likely contenders and both have been investigated. However, as Glover (1992, p. 609) points out:

> ... there is, as yet, little direct evidence for a role for these hormones in postnatal mental disturbance. No one has yet found that sufferers have clearly different absolute levels on any particular day to non-sufferers.

Harris (1994) reviews a number of studies on the effects of oestrogen and progesterone and concludes that although there is some support for the use of oestrogen in treating women with postnatal depression, the evidence for the importance of these hormones in causing or treating PND remains weak. Progesterone has been used as a treatment, but no double blind trials have been undertaken to prove its effectiveness.

Cortisol has been linked with depression at other times of life and in certain illnesses such as Cushing's syndrome (Harris, 1994). However, once again studies have failed to show a relationship between cortisol levels and postpartum depression. Some tentative links have been shown with b-endorphin, but once again findings remain weak. Other biochemical changes have also been studied, but researchers have found it impossible to draw firm or consistent conclusions because many other factors can influence these changes.

Finally, Harris (1993) believes that, 'women who have episodes of postpartum thyroiditis and who are positive for thyroid antibodies are prone to episodes of postpartum depression' (p. 288). Harris and his co-workers have done a large amount of research on this but it only explains a small percentage of women who become depressed following birth and leaves other cases of PND with no obvious cause.

Recently it has been argued that there might be two populations of women who experience PND. One for whom the depression is specifically related to the emotional demands of motherhood and another for whom the birth is either unrelated or a non-specific stressor. Cooper and Murray (1995) studied three groups of women following birth, thirty-four who had depression following birth without having experienced depression previously (de novo), twenty-one who became postnatally depressed but who had suffered from depression in the past and a group of forty psychiatrically well women. They hypothesised that the de novo subjects would be more likely to become depressed following subsequent birth than other groups. The evidence supported this hypothesis, as 41% of the women who had experienced first onset of PND had a later depression twelve weeks after the birth of another child. This was compared with 12% of the control group and 18% of those with recurrent depression. Although Cooper and Murray suggest that these results support a biological explanation of PND, it seems equally possible that the de novo group could simply be experiencing more difficulty with the transition to motherhood than the other groups and, despite advocating a biological explanation, they acknowledge:

> *... despite extensive research into steroid hormones in women during the puerperium, no firm evidence has emerged linking these hormones to the development of postnatal depression.*
>
> (Cooper and Murray, 1995 p. 194)

Even dyed-in-the-wool biologically-orientated writers are beginning to acknowledge that it is difficult to be dogmatic about a biological cause of postnatal depression when it continues to elude researchers.

> *... there must be a delicate balance and interaction between biological and environmental stressors in the context of pregnancy. This means that a global approach is necessary when dealing with the various mental states which occur particularly after delivery, ie. attention should be given to each and every potential cause of mental disorder not excluding, or only concentrating on, the biological factors.*
>
> (Harris, 1996, p. 35)

Finally, Hendrick *et al* (1998) carried out an analysis of many studies of hormonal involvement in postnatal depression. They looked at the role of progesterone, oestrogen, prolactin, cortisol, oxytocin, thyroid and vasopressin and concluded that there was no firm evidence that linked any of these hormones to the aetiology of postnatal depression.

What can we conclude then about biological causes of postnatal depression? As this brief review of the literature has shown, a straightforward biological explanation has not yet been found and there are many criticisms that can be made of the research. For example, other aspects of postnatal depression argue against it. If PND was a reaction to changes in biochemistry or hormone levels following birth, one would expect all women to suffer from it. (Chalmers and Chalmers, 1986). After all, similar biological changes occur in all women, if this were the explanation why do some women succumb and not others. Similarly, if biological factors alone were the cause, you would not expect such a wide variation in time of onset. How can hormone changes influence a woman three or even six months after she has given birth? By this time any biological changes due to the birth should have normalised.

Another criticism is the old problem of attributing causality. Although some research has shown a relationship between various biological factors and postnatal depression, this alone does not demonstrate that the one causes the other. It could be the other way round, that depression creates biochemical and other changes in the body, or alternatively, it could be that the apparent relationship is spurious and there is no meaningful connection between the two things at all.

What interests me most about biological explanations of PND is why researchers continue to persist with this line of investigation when the search for a straightforward biological cause of postpartum depression has been so fruitless. The most common justification given for the research, is that once a cause has been found then treatment can be given and so alleviate the suffering. Presumably this treatment would be in the form of a simple pill or injection. This would certainly be an easy way of dealing with mental anguish and other factors, which might be causing women to become depressed, could be ignored. It would be cost-effective too; a course of pills would no doubt be cheaper than counselling.

Another explanation for the persistence in seeking for a biological cause is the long medical tradition of believing that women's reproductive abilities are linked to their mental well being. This can be traced back centuries to the time of Hippocrates when women's madness was thought to be due to the womb wandering around the body (Ussher, 1992a). The idea flourished in the Victorian period when all manner of female ailments were laid at the door of the reproductive cycle.

> *The monthly activity of the ovaries... has a notable effect upon the mind and body; wherefore it may become an important cause of mental and physical derangement... It is a matter of common experience in asylums, that exacerbations of insanity often take place at menstrual periods.*

([Maudsley, 1873, p. 88] quoted in Ussher, 1992b)

Hormones are argued to be at the root of pre-menstrual syndrome affecting a woman's concentration, making her feel emotional, and even affecting her ability to drive. All kinds of mental 'symptoms' have been put down to menopause, ranging from inability to concentrate to depression. Being a psychologist and possibly deemed not to have an in-depth grasp of biology, perhaps I am over-simplifying the situation, but I often wonder why the biological mechanisms that exist to regulate a woman's ability to reproduce should affect her emotional well being? Where is the logic in it?

Reducing women's mental anguish to her 'raging hormones' certainly side-steps issues about women's place in society. Maybe it is easier to reduce women's distress to a simple biochemical imbalance, which can be corrected with appropriate treatment, rather than confronting what it is really about. Certainly the biological approach to postnatal depression ignores all the other factors in a woman's life that may be contributing to her mental distress at the point of becoming a mother.

Perhaps I am being too harsh here on those who persist in seeking a biological explanation for postnatal depression. Some time in the future maybe a link between hormones and emotions will be discovered and the pathways by which they interact upon each other will be better understood. But this will not be a simple relationship of cause and effect, we will have to understand how biological and psychosocial factors *interact* if we are to gain a real understanding of why some women experience postnatal depression while others do not.

Psychosocial explanations

Some researchers, critical of the biological approach have argued that PND cannot simply be explained in terms of biological factors and have looked for causes located in personal psychology and the social environment of the individual. Pitt (1968) was perhaps the earliest researcher to argue that postnatal depression was due to what he called 'non-specific stress' (Watson *et al*, 1984). A study by Brown and Harris conducted in 1978 on a community of women living in London, had demonstrated that depression appeared to be more common in those who had experienced certain life events, such as death of their own mother before the age of eleven, having three children at home under the age of five and having no one in whom they felt that they could confide. It seemed possible that similar 'risk' factors might be found to be related to depression that occurred specifically in the postpartum and it has been argued that the weight of evidence so far points to a psychological/social causation:

> *There is common ground between all studies so far that the main aetiological factors are to be found in the psychological and social domain.*

> (Kumar, 1994, p. 256)

Once again the research findings are not straightforward and such a positive conclusion as that given above is perhaps premature. Although it appears logical to assume that depression will occur in mothers who have difficult life circumstances, there is a lack of clarity in the conclusions of the research that has been carried out so far. Almost every study that you look at finds that some risk factors are related to depression, but the range of factors reported are wide and seem to vary from study to study. A useful summary of studies carried out in Western Europe and North America may be found in Richards (1990). This author reports that women who have a poor relationship with their partner have a greater risk of becoming depressed postnatally. Poor quality social support and the lack of a confidante for the mother were other vulnerability factors found by most but not all of the studies reviewed by Richards. Adverse social circumstances and life events have been linked to an increased susceptibility to PND. Low income has also been reported as a vulnerability factor in some studies.

More recent studies have reported other risk factors. For example, in a study conducted on 217 women, Hannah *et al* (1992) found that in the first week postpartum, high scores on the Edinburgh Postnatal Depression scale were related to bottle feeding, delivery by Caesarean section, low birth weight of the baby and a more difficult delivery than expected; but by the sixth postnatal week only bottle feeding and delivery by Caesarean section were still related to PND. A study by Murray *et al* (1995) using the EPDS to screen for depression in the postnatal period found that high scores were related to two factors, namely: occupational instability and a poor relationship with the woman's own mother. Warner *et al* (1996), studied 2375 women and found that at six to eight weeks postpartum, four variables were related to a high EPDS score, these included unplanned pregnancy, bottle feeding, unemployment in the mother and unemployment in the mother's partner. Seguin (1999) has shown that low socioeconomic status and chronic stressors, such as maternal health problems and lack of money for basic needs are associated with postnatal depression. A study by De Mier *et al* (2000) has linked postnatal emotional distress with the gestational age of the baby, Apgar ratings and birth complications. Previous experience of sexual abuse is also a risk factor. Women who have been sexually abused report significantly higher levels of depressive symptomatology following birth (Benedict *et al*, 1999).

Beck (2001) carried out a meta-analysis of eighty-four studies published in the 1990s and found that there were thirteen significant predictors of postnatal depression. These included prenatal depression, childcare stress, self-esteem, prenatal anxiety, life stress, social support, marital relationship, history of previous depression, infant temperament, maternity blues, marital status, socioeconomic status and unplanned or unwanted pregnancy.

Although this is by no means an exhaustive review of the literature, it can be seen that there is a wide range of so-called 'risk factors' that have been identified. *Table 9.2* summarises the risk factors that have been implicated in the studies discussed above.

Table 9.2: Summary of psychosocial risk factors and researchers

Risk factor	Researcher
Poor relationship with partner	Richards, 1990
Lack of a confidante	Richards, 1990
Poor quality social support	Richards, 1990
Adverse social circumstances	Richards, 1990
Low income	Seguin, 1999
Delivery by Caesarean section	Hannah *et al*, 1992
Occupational instability	Murray *et al*, 1995
Poor relationship with own mother	Murray *et al*, 1995
Unplanned pregnancy	Warner *et al*, 1996
Unemployment in self or partner	Warner *et al*, 1996
Past history of depressive illness	Beck, 2001
Gestational age of baby, birth complications	De Mier *et al*, 2000
Chronic stressors	Seguin, 1999; O'Hara and Swain, 1996
Low socioeconomic status	Seguin, 1999; O'Hara and Swain, 1996
Bottle feeding	Hannah, 1992; Warner, 1996
Experience of sexual abuse	Benedict *et al*, 1999
Ambivalence about the pregnancy	Beck, 2001

Such a wide range of factors have been reported that it calls into question how useful this concept is for identifying women who are at risk. Most researchers justify the continuing search for risk factors with the argument that if they can be identified then women who are most likely to become postnatally depressed can be recognised early and given medical help and counselling. In reality, there are so many risk factors that it becomes almost impossible to predict who will suffer from postnatal depression and who will not, as many, if not all pregnant women would have experienced at least some of the risk factors that have been listed in *Table 9.2*.

O'Hara and Swain (1996) carried out a meta-analysis of

fifty-nine studies, all of which met fairly stringent criteria for inclusion in their study. Altogether 12,810 women were reviewed and it was concluded that the prevalence rate was 13%. These authors believe that on the basis of their analysis they can produce a picture of the 'prototypical pregnant woman at risk for postpartum depression'. It is worth quoting this at some length.

> *She is most likely to occupy a lower social stratum but also women representing middle and upper strata will be abundantly represented. She is very likely to have experienced life stressors during pregnancy and may have had a more difficult than normal pregnancy or delivery. She will be experiencing marital difficulties and experience her partner as providing little in the way of social support. Compounding the life stress will be her perception that others in her social network are not particularly supportive of her. Finally, her history will show evidence of psychopathology, in most cases major depression or dysthymia and she will show evidence of being at least mildly depressed, and excessively worried.*

(p. 53)

Apart from the fact that I find this description extremely patronising, I wonder if this kind of stereotyping is at all helpful for either the clinician or midwife? Does it really enable us to predict the woman who will be depressed when she comes into the antenatal clinic or when we see her on the ward after delivery? There are so many possible combinations of potential risk factors that we would need to have in depth knowledge of every individual woman before being able to make a judgement about her likelihood of suffering from PND. The use of such stereotypes might also blind us to women who did not fit the categories but who nevertheless became depressed. The middle class woman with a comfortable home and no obvious risk factors could easily be overlooked.

Does postnatal depression exist in all cultures or is it specific to Western Europe and North America? If postnatal depression is caused by psychosocial factors then it is possible that women from different cultures would be either more or less likely to suffer from PND depending on the way that they are treated following birth. Those who believe that PND is caused by psychosocial factors argue that different social mores will mean that women in some cultures will be enabled to adapt to motherhood more easily than others and will be protected from postnatal depression. Stern and Kruckman (1983) and Cox (1988, 1996) have both argued that PND would be less likely to occur in cultures where there were more formal 'rites of passage' following birth. They suggest that depression is common in Western industrialised cultures because women are cut adrift from the help given by the traditional extended family and are simply left to cope with a difficult life transition on their own. Cox argued that in such cultures, there is very little support for women once they have left hospital; they are given no special treatment, accorded no privileged status and are expected to return to normal life as quickly as possible. In cultures where women are treated differently after birth, where they are cared for for longer periods and allowed to rest, postnatal depression will be less common because these different social practices give them the chance to recover physically, and psychologically make the transition to motherhood.

To test Cox's theory, Moon-Park and Dimigen (1995) compared a sample of Scottish and Korean women. Traditional practices in Korea appear to provide the kind of postpartum support that Cox suggests will help women to avoid postnatal depression. Women are cared for by their parents or parents-in-law for a period of twenty-one days after birth. During this time visitors are kept away, the mother is allowed to rest and is given special foods that are thought to help her return to full strength. At the end of this time, they are expected to return to their own home and normal duties. The Scottish women in contrast, stayed in hospital for only a few days, after which time they returned home and carried on with their lives. Contrary to expectations, these researchers, using the Beck Depression Inventory, found that the Korean sample demonstrated more symptoms of depression than the Scottish mothers did. This finding could have been due to the fact that the interview took place just before the end of the three-week period, when the Korean women had to face a return home and withdrawal of support, whereas the Scottish sample had already had several weeks in which to adjust to their new routines. However, it did not support Cox's hypothesis.

While the majority of studies on PND have been carried out in North America and Western Europe there are an increasing number of studies being carried out on women from other cultures, however it is often difficult to make accurate comparisons (Kumar, 1994). Ghubash and Abou-Saleh (1997) carried out research on a sample of 102 women from Dubai, in the United Arab Emirates. Like Moon-Park and Dimigen, these researchers found similar prevalence rates to those in Europe and North America. Yamashito (2000) also found similar prevalence rates in a sample of Japanese women. Cooper *et al* (1999) studied 147 women in South Africa and recorded somewhat different results. The prevalence rate of postnatal depression was 4.7% markedly higher than that reported in many other cultures. Dankner *et al* (2000) looking at a sample of Jewish women in Jerusalem also found that the prevalence rate was higher among Orthodox Jews. In fact, from the cross-cultural studies that can be accurately compared it seems that there are no major differences in prevalence of postnatal depression to be found (Kumar 1994), indicating that different cultural practices do not have a major impact on negative emotional reactions in the postpartum. The prevalence rate in the countries that have been studied so far is, with a few exceptions, remarkably consistent. This could be seen as evidence supportive of a biological cause of postnatal depression. On the other hand, it could also indicate that there is something about becoming a mother that causes some women to react with depression.

In conclusion, while psychosocial explanations of postnatal depression do at least acknowledge that women become depressed in the postnatal period for reasons that are complex and have more to do with their social circumstances and experience of motherhood than with their hormones, there are still criticisms that can be made of the approach. Researchers who look for psychosocial risk factors are using the same rather simplistic and reductionist models as those looking for biological causes, and they make similar assumptions about causality. Both approaches presume that PND has some under-lying cause which, if identified, will explain the emotional response, and both regard postnatal depression as an abnormal reaction to motherhood.

As with the biological explanations discussed earlier, it seems that researchers have found it impossible to identify any psycho-social risk factors that are consistently related to postnatal depression. This means that we are no nearer building up a picture of which individuals are most likely to succumb to depression in the postpartum. We should therefore question whether the continuing search for 'psychosocial risk factors' is at all helpful to women who have postnatal depression.

The two approaches share similar difficulties about causality; as we have seen many risk factors are related to PND, but we are no nearer knowing whether any of these actually cause it. It could simply be that the risk factors that have been identified in the various studies become more salient to people when they are feeling depressed. For example, if you are experiencing negative emotions after having a baby perhaps you feel the lack of a confidante more acutely, and attach significance to this. We all have a tendency to look actively for reasons to interpret our feelings; if mothers are unable to explain their depression in terms of their adjustment to motherhood, they might well look for other explanations that are more acceptable to them.

So, where does all this lead? We have considered both biological and psychosocial explanations of postnatal depression in some detail, and have found them wanting. Despite many studies neither approach has been able to explain conclusively what causes postnatal depression and we are no nearer being able to predict who will experience it, or how it should best be treated. We know that there are psychosocial factors that are related to it, and we feel that there could possibly be a biological cause if only we were skilful enough to find it, but we remain uncertain. Meanwhile there are many women who continue to suffer from depression, feeling unhappy, guilty and frequently unable to tell anyone what they are going through. Is there a different way of looking at the problem that might be more helpful to women? I think that there is an alternative that avoids some of the difficulties that we have discussed with the other approaches and is ultimately a better explanation of what is happening to women in the postpartum period. This approach recognises that motherhood is both culturally defined and requires substantial personal adjustment that each woman will cope with differently. It also takes individual experience into account and prioritises what the transition to motherhood means.

An alternative way of looking at postnatal depression

It is impossible to remove postnatal depression from the social context in which it occurs; and despite the fact that women in the twenty-first century are more liberated than their mothers or grandmothers were, there are still difficulties inherent in being female in a society that is largely dominated by male values. Feminist researchers argue that women become depressed postnatally, neither because of their hormones, nor because of so-called risk factors (although these may play a part) but because of the conflicting demands made on them by their position in society (Ussher, 1992a). Mothering is a role that, on the one hand is revered, but on the other is given little status (Phoenix and Woollett, 1991) and after giving birth some women find themselves socially isolated and unsupported, feeling they have lost any individual identity. When this loss of identity is coupled with the demands of constant caring it seems hardly surprising that women experience depression. As Ussher points out:

> *The 'depression' may actually be a normal part of the experience of motherhood, even an adaptive process allowing the woman to grieve for her lost self and to make the transition to motherhood.*

(Ussher, 1992b, p. 50)

Another aspect of modern life that may exacerbate the difficulties experienced by women in the postnatal period is that we live in a society where the needs of the individual are valued to such an extent that we attach great importance to pursuing our own goals. Unlike previous generations, we think that everyone has the right to be happy about themselves, their job and their lifestyle and so on. In terms of human society this way of thinking has only become possible at a point in history where society is relatively stable and individuals are not struggling every day simply with the task of surviving. We now have leisure to consider and indulge our own needs. I do not mean this to sound puritanical (although I am aware that it probably does), I merely wish to suggest that for some women the transition to motherhood may be more difficult now than it has ever been. Modern women are (rightly) able to engage in activities that were previously only open to men. Effective contraception means that we can choose when, and how many children we have and we no longer see bearing the next generation as our major role in life; we actively pursue our own careers and interests. By contrast, motherhood as it is constructed in Western society often demands that for a period of time at least, women suspend their own identities whilst caring for their infant twenty-four hours a day. They may find that they have no time to engage in activities that were previously highly valued. Even everyday activities can become problematic; as one depressed mother of a young baby once said to me, 'I can't even go to the shop to buy a bag of potatoes now, without it becoming a major expedition'.

Given all this, and as it is possible to find reasons why women might find motherhood depressing, why do we continue to treat PND as if it were abnormal? There is a persisting view that pervades virtually all the literature, that postnatal depression is a **pathological** response to motherhood; because it is abnormal, there must be some underlying biological or psychosocial cause. This view is odd because in other cases where people experience an event that strongly influences their life, such as divorce, redundancy or bereavement a period of depression and personal readjustment is expected and is certainly not treated as unusual. Why is it that becoming a mother should be treated so differently from other life changing events?

Many feminists would argue that the answer to this question can be found in the cultural discourse that sees motherhood as 'natural' and the birth of a baby as a 'happy' time. The belief that PND is abnormal can only persist because we see it in the context of an ideology that states that women are supposed to love being mothers and take to it like ducks to water; when they become depressed they are considered unusual. We are all strongly influenced by this view of motherhood, doctors, midwives, psychologists and, of course, women themselves. When women have the belief that mothering should come naturally it is very difficult for them to admit to being depressed but it is possible to look at it in a different way. If the transition to motherhood is seen as a significant life change that requires physical and psychological adaptation then a period of depression in the postnatal period simply becomes one stage in the process of adjusting to a new life situation.

If we consider the transition to motherhood we can see that there are many changes after birth that require some degree of physical and psychological adaptation and could potentially contribute to depression.

1. Women can never be prepared for the impact that motherhood has on their lives. Everything changes, even simple tasks that were once taken for granted, may no longer be easy to accomplish.
2. Birth may be more traumatic than anticipated and women need time to recover emotionally (just like the post-operative patients in Levy's study [1994]). However, this is often difficult when coupled with the demands of caring for a baby.
3. It is well documented that any major lifestyle change, even a positive one, requires a period of adaptation that may involve a phase of feeling depressed. Why should becoming a mother be any different?
4. In cultures where the nuclear family is the norm, women may receive little practical help and caring for an infant twenty-four hours a day can be overwhelming and physically exhausting.

5.   Women themselves expect that they will be able to cope with motherhood and may be astonished to find that they cannot.

Paula Nicolson (1989, 1990) has suggested that it is more helpful to see depression following birth as a reaction to loss. Although the images of new motherhood that abound in society imply that women have all to gain, in the light of the previous discussion it can be seen that this is not necessarily so. As she points out:

> *Having a baby... requires a total change of role; it involves a change in body image and loss of former psychological identity; it affects the balance of relationships and power inside and outside the home and orientation to work/ career (even if the woman returns to work) and subjects frequently report they have less in common with old friends.*

(Nicolson, 1990, p. 694)

We know that adaptation to any kind of loss involves a period of depression, therefore such an explanation appears to be a more powerful way of explaining many of the aspects of PND that have refused to fall within the remit of the biological or psychosocial standpoints. To review these briefly, postnatal depression does not have a clear time of onset, it can occur at any time in the first postnatal year. No consistent biological causal factors or psychosocial risk factors have been found, although many have been suggested. The symptoms are many and diverse and it is impossible to know who will be most susceptible to becoming depressed. Nicolson's model neatly answers many of these problems by making the prediction that what causes postnatal depression is a response to loss that will be experienced uniquely by every individual. Whether a woman becomes depressed will depend on her own psycho- logical coping strategies and on how she sees the life changes brought about by motherhood. For some women it will be the loss of control experienced at the birth or inability to breast feed that may be significant. For others it could be the loss of body image, others may find it difficult to cope with losing their job, others may grieve the loss of valued activities. The list is endless and infinitely variable from one woman to another.

Social support comes into this too. While all women share the emotional upheaval of becoming a mother, some will have strong emotional support from significant others to help them get through this difficult period while others may not. Perhaps this explains why lack of a confidante has been one of the few consistent psychosocial explanations that have emerged from the literature. If you are grieving and feeling sad, it helps to talk to someone who is sympathetic and tries to understand your situation.

If Nicolson's ideas about postnatal depression being caused by adjusting to a difficult life event are correct, then one might predict that fathers too could be susceptible to depression following the birth of a child. Although there have not been many studies carried out, some preliminary investigations indicate that depression is not uncommon in new fathers. Ballard and Davies (1996) found that more than 10% of fathers experience depression. It is still not clear whether new fathers are more at risk than men in the general population, but in their study they did find that having an unsupportive relationship and being unemployed both seemed to be related. This study lends some weight to the argument that we should stop searching for biological or psychosocial risk factors and begin to look at what new motherhood means to women. Only then will we begin to understand an individual's response and stand any chance of predicting whether they will experience depression.

Explaining postnatal depression in terms of a model of loss is more helpful than either the biological or psychosocial models because of its ability to explain individual variation among women. It also explains why women do not necessarily experience depression with every pregnancy and why it occurs in all cultures. The experience of becoming a mother will be different in different societies but, whatever society you look at, it always involves a major change in a woman's life.

I have only given a brief account of Nicolson's ideas about postnatal depression here. If you are interested in reading more you might like to read her book published in 1998. She has also written an excellent book suitable for mothers.

Although Nicolson's model of loss explains many of the enigmatic aspects of postnatal depression, it may be argued that its major weakness is that it does not allow health professionals to predict easily who will experience PND. This is a valid criticism. The only way of knowing who is depressed is to listen to individuals and hear what they are saying about how they are coping with the transition to motherhood and what changes are significant to them. This may be perceived as impossibly time-consuming by those who would like to be able to use a simple screening device to identify women at risk. In practice, it is what health professionals have to do because we still do not have a simple way of identifying women at risk of depression. Although in many studies the EPDS is now used as a screening tool, it can only be used to identify women once they have become depressed and may, in fact, miss many women who are only mildly depressed or anxious to disguise their symptoms.

It would help if we stopped expecting all women to respond to motherhood with happy contentment and began to accept that some will find the adjustment difficult. This is what we do with other major life changes such as redundancy or bereavement and we do not consider screening people who are 'at risk' of becoming depressed following divorce. It is accepted that it is a major life change and some people will respond by becoming depressed. If attitudes changed then there would not be such a stigma attached to postnatal depression and more women would feel able to approach health professionals for help.

What can the midwife do to help?

I hope that this chapter has helped you to see that there is a great deal that a midwife could do to help women to cope with depression following birth. Education is essential to help women to see:

- that postnatal depression is a common reaction to birth
- that it is not to be feared
- that it is an understandable response to a life event that may require a great deal of personal adjustment.

If women could come to understand PND in this way more would come forward for help and, ironically, it could reduce the duration of depression for many women too. Sufferers of postpartum depression often stay depressed for longer than necessary simply because they are afraid to admit their feelings to anyone (Mauthner, 1997). There are several reasons for this: some women fear that their babies will be removed from them, especially if they have had negative feelings about them; others are ashamed because they feel that they are not supposed to be depressed and should be happy; while others know that there is something wrong but do not report the symptoms because they think that it is quite normal to feel like this after childbirth (Whitton *et al*, 1996).

Antenatal classes are an obvious place to encourage women to talk about postnatal depression and consider what is known about it. When I talk to midwives they often say that it is difficult to discuss negative aspects of pregnancy and motherhood during antenatal classes. I accept that it is not always easy to raise negative issues, but there is no evidence that this causes distress (Cox, 1989) and the potential benefits to women would outweigh any slight negative effects. If women were encouraged to consider ways that their lives could change after birth, they might be helped to see that many personal adjustments were required. This could then be used as a starting point to suggest that a period of depression is a reaction to motherhood that could be experienced by some women. Approaching the topic in this way might enable women to see postnatal depression, not as a stigma but as part of the process of adapting to a new lifestyle. If the stigma were removed and women with depression could stop seeing themselves as abnormal, they would be far more likely to seek help earlier and suffer the depression for a shorter period. The spin-offs for the mother and her family would be enormous.

Although as a midwife you have only limited contact with a woman once she has given birth, it is helpful to know what the options are for treatment once postnatal depression has occurred. There is now considerable evidence to show that counselling is effective, it can be given either individually or in groups (Elliott *et al*, 1988; Nicolson, 1989; Leverton, 1991) and appears to be as effective in treating postnatal depression as fluoxetine, an antidepressant drug (Appleby *et al*, 1997). Holden *et al* (1989) found that if health visitors spent half an hour a week listening to a mother's problems in a supportive and empathetic way, it was helpful for at least a third of the mothers in their sample who were suffering from depression and no additional treatment was needed. Midwives could do this too in the nine or ten days that they see women postnatally. Listening to women in this period could also alert health professionals to women who were becoming depressed. This information could be passed on to health visitors and GPs. Ultimately, as Cox suggests, this brief intervention could save time for the health professionals and reduce the incidence of depression.

In the more severe cases of postnatal depression, counselling may not be adequate and some form of medication may be necessary. Hospitalisation and more specialised psychiatric help may be needed in cases of puerperal psychosis. There are a few mother and baby units throughout the country where mothers can stay with their babies and receive specialised psychiatric help, but the provision is woefully inadequate and cannot possibly treat all the women who are in need of support. Clearly, there needs to be more provision made in this area of health care.

In short, education and counselling are both effective tools that could be used together to help women overcome postnatal depression.

Education should help women and society at large to take a more realistic view of motherhood and recognise that it is a major life change that will require adjustment and may involve some grieving for aspects of a former lifestyle that have been lost. Listening to what women are saying about their experiences of motherhood enables them to express any distress that they may be feeling in a context where their emotions are accepted and they are not made to feel that they are abnormal or unnatural mothers. Together they might help women come to terms with postnatal depression and recover from it more quickly.

References

Albright A (1993) Postpartum depression: an overview. *J Counselling Development* **7**: 316–20

Appleby L, Kumar C, Warner R (1996) Perinatal psychiatry. *Int Rev Psychiatry* **8**: 5–7

Appleby L, Warner R, Whitton A, Faragher B (1997) A controlled study of fluoxetine and cognitive-behavioural counselling in the treatment of postnatal depression. *Br Med J* **314**: 932–6

Appleby L, Mortenson PB, Faragher EB (1998) Suicide and other causes of mortality after post partum psychiatric admission. *Br J Psychiatry* **173**: 209–11

Armstrong KL, Van Haeringen AR, Dadds MR, Cash R (1998) Sleep deprivation or postnatal depression in later infancy: separating the chicken from the egg. *J Paediatr Child Health* **34**(3): 260–2

Ballard C, Davies R (1996) Postnatal depression in fathers. *Int Rev Psychiatry* **8**: 65–71

Beck CT (2001) Predictors of postpartum depression: an update. *Nurs Res* **50**(5): 275–85

Bedford A, Foulds G (1978) *Delusions-symptoms-states. State of Anxiety and Depression (Manual)*. National Foundation for Educational Research, Windsor

Beck AT, Ward CH, Mendelson M *et al* (1961) An inventory for measuring depression. *Arch Gen Psychiatry* **4**: 561–71

Benedict MI, Paine LL, Paine LA, Brandt D, Stallings R (1999) The association of childhood sexual abuse with depressive symptoms during pregnancy and selected pregnancy outcomes. *Child Abuse Negl* **23**(7): 659–70

Brockington I (1996) *Motherhood and Mental Health*. Oxford University Press, Oxford

Brown GW, Harris T (1978) *Social Origins of Depression*. Tavistock, London

Catalbiano NJ, Catalbiano ML (1996) Relationship between exhaustion and postnatal depression. *Psychol Rep* **79**: 225–6

Chalmers BE, Chalmers BM (1986) Postpartum depression: a revised perspective. *J Psychosom Obstet Gynaecol* **5**: 93–105

Cooper PJ, Campbell EA, Day A, Kennerley H, Bond A (1988) Non-psychotic psychiatric disorder after childbirth. A prospective study of prevalence, incidence, course and nature. *Br J Psychiatry* **152**: 799–806

Cooper PJ, Murray L (1995) Course and recurrence of postnatal depression — evidence for the specificity of the diagnostic concept. *Br J Psychiatry* **166**: 191–5

Cooper PJ, Tomlinson M, Swartz L, Woolgar M, Murray L, Moltena C (1999) Post-partum depression and the mother-infant relationship in a South African peri-urban settlement. *Br J Psychiatry* **175**: 554–8

Cox JL, Connor Y, Kendell RE (1982) Prospective study of the psychiatric disorders of childbirth. *Br J Psychiatry* **140**: 111–17

Cox JL, Holden JM, Sagovsky R (1987) Detection of postnatal depression: Development of the 10-item Edinburgh Postnatal Depression Scale. *Br J Psychiatry* **150**: 782–6

Cox JL (1988) The life events of childbirth: Sociocultural aspects of childbirth. In: Kumar R, Brockington IF, eds. *Motherhood and Mental Illness 2: Causes and consequences*. Wright, London: 64–77

Cox JL (1989) Can postnatal depression be prevented? *Midwife, Health Visitor and Community Nurse* **25**(8): 326–9

Cox JL (1996) Perinatal mental disorder — a cultural approach. *Int Rev Psychiatry* **8**: 9–16

Dankner R, Goldberg RP, Fishc RZ, Crum RM (2000) Cultural elements of postpartum depression. A study of 327 Jewish Jerusalem women. *J Reprod Med* **45**(2): 97–104

De Mier RL, Hynan MT, Hatfield RF, Varner MW, Harris HB, Manniello RL (2000) A measurement model of perinatal stressors: identifying risk for postnatal emotional distress in mothers of high-risk infants. *J Clin Psychol* **56**(1): 89–100

Elliott SA, Sanjack M, Leverton TJ (1988) Parents groups in pregnancy: A preventive intervention for postnatal depression? In: Gottlieb BJ, ed. *Marshalling Social Support*. Sage, Newbury Park, California

Ghubash R, Abou-Saleh MT (1997) Post-partum psychiatric illness in Arab culture: prevalence and psychosocial correlates. *Br J Psychiatry* **171**: 65–8

Glover V (1992) Do biochemical factors play a part in postnatal depression? *Prog Neuro-psychopharmacol Bio Psychiat* **16**: 605–15

Goldberg DP, Cooper B, Eastwood MR *et al* (1970) A standardised psychiatric interview for use in community surveys. *Br J Social Preventative Med* **24**: 18–23

Goldberg DP (1972) *The detection of psychiatric illness by questionnaire. Maudsley Monograph 21*. Oxford University Press, Oxford

Gotlib IH, Whiffen VE, Mount JH, Milne K, Cordy NI (1989) Prevalence rates and demographic characteristics associated with depression in pregnancy and the postpartum. *J Consult Clin Psychol* **57**(2): 269–74

Jackson R (1994) *Mothers Who Leave London*. Pandora, London

Jebali C (1993) A feminist perspective on postnatal depression. *Health Visitor* **66**(2): 59–60

Jennings KD, Ross S, Popper S, Elmore M (1999) Thoughts of harming infants in depressed and non-depressed mothers. *J Affect Disord* **54**(1–2): 21–8

Hannah P, Adams D, Lee A, Glover V, Sandler M (1992) Links between early post-partum mood and post-natal depression. *Br J Psychiatry* **160**: 777–80

Harding JJ (1989) Postpartum psychiatric disorders. *Compr Psychiatry* **30**: 109–12

Harris B (1993) A hormonal component to postnatal depression. *Br J Psychiatry* **163**: 403–5

Harris B (1994) Biological and hormonal aspects of postpartum depressed mood. Working towards strategies for prophylaxis and treatment. Special issue. Depression. *Br J Psychiatry* **164**: 288–92

Harris B (1996) Hormonal aspects of PND. *Int Rev Psychiatry* **8**: 27–36

Hendrick V, Atshuler LL, Suri R (1998) Hormonal changes in the postpartum and implication for postpartum depression. *Psychosom* **39**(2): 93–101

Holden JM, Sagovsky R, Cox JL (1989) Counselling in a general practice setting: controlled intervention in treatment of postnatal depression. *Br Med J* **298**: 223–6

Jebali CA (1993) A feminist perspective on postnatal depression. *Health Visitor* **66**(2): 59–60

Kumar R, Robson KM (1984) A prospective study of emotional disorders in childbearing women. *Br J Psychiatry* **144**: 35–47

Kumar R (1994) Postnatal mental illness: a transcultural perspective. *Soc Psychiatry Psychiatr Epidemiol* **29**(6): 250–64

Lavender T, Walkinshaw SA (1998) Can midwives reduce postpartum psychological morbidity? A randomized trial. *Birth* **25**(4): 215–9

Leverton TJ (1991) Group treatment for depressed mothers of pre-school children. *Matern Child Health* **10**: 332–4

Levy V (1994) The maternity blues in postpartum women and postoperative patients. In: Robinson S, Thomas AM, eds. *Midwives, Research and Childbirth*. Vol 3. Chapman and Hall, London: 147–74

Mauthner NS (1997) Postnatal depression: how can midwives help? *Midwifery* **13**(4): 163–71

McIntosh J (1993) Postpartum depression: women's help-seeking behaviour and perceptions of cause. *J Adv Nurs* **18**: 178–84

Moon-Park EH, Dimigon G (1995) A cross cultural comparison: postnatal depression in Korean and Scottish mothers. *Int J Psychol in the Orient* **38**(3): 199–207

Murray D, Cox JL, Chapman G, Jones P (1995) Childbirth: Life event or start of a long-term difficulty? Further data from the Stoke-on-Trent controlled study of postnatal depression. *Br J Psychiatry* **166**: 595–600

Nicolson P (1989) Counselling women with postnatal depression: complications from recent qualitative research. *Counsel Psychol Quarterly* **2**(2): 123–32

Nicolson P (1998) *Postnatal Depression: Psychology, science and the transition to motherhood*. Routledge, London

Nicolson P (1990) Understanding postnatal depression: a mother-centred approach. *J Adv Nurs* **15**: 689–95

Nicolson P (2001) *PND — Facing the Paradox of Loss, Happiness and Motherhood*. Wiley, London

Oakley A (1979) The baby blues. *New Society* **4**: 11–12

Oakley A, Chamberlain G (1981) Medical and social factors in postpartum depression. *J Obstet Gynaecol* **1**: 182–7

O'Hara MW, Neunaber DJ, Zekoski EM (1984) A prospective study of postpartum depression: prevalence, course and predictive factors. *J Abnormal Psychol* **93**: 158–71

O'Hara MW, Swain AM (1996) Rates and risk of postpartum depression — a meta-analysis. *Int Rev Psychiatry* **8**: 37–54

Paykel ES, Emms EM, Fletcher J, Rassaby ES (1980) Life events and social support in puerperal depression. *Br J Psychiatry* **136**: 339–46

Pfuhlmann B, Franzek E, Beckmann H, Stober G (1999) Long-term course outcome of severe postpartum psychiatric disorders. *Psychopathol* **32**(4): 192–202

Phoenix A, Woollett A (1991) Motherhood: social construction, politics and psychology. In: Phoenix A, Woollette A, Lloyd E, eds. *Motherhood: Meanings, practices and ideologies.* Sage, London

Pitt B (1968) 'Atypical depression' following childbirth. *Br J Psychiatry* **114**: 1325–35

Richards JP (1990) Postnatal depression: a review of recent literature. *Br J Gen Pract* **40**: 472–6

Seguin L, Potrin L, St-Denis M, Loiselle J (1999) Depressive symptoms in the late postpartum among low socioeconomic status women. *Birth* **26**(3): 157–63

Stern G, Kruckman L (1983) Multi-disciplinary perspectives on post-partum depression: An anthropological critique. *Soc Sci Med* **17**: 1027–41

Ussher J (1992a) Research and theory related to female reproduction: Implications for clinical psychology. *Br J Clin Psychol* **31**: 129–51

Ussher J (1992b) Reproductive rhetoric and the blaming of the body. In: Nicolson P, Ussher J, eds. *The Psychology of Women's Health and Health Care.* Macmillan Press, Basingstoke

Warner R, Appleby L, Whitton A, Faragher B (1996) Demographic and obstetric risk factors for postnatal psychiatric morbidity. *Br J Psychiatry* **168**: 607–11

Watson JP, Elliott SA, Rugg AJ, Brough DI (1984) Psychiatric disorder and the first postnatal year. *Br J Psychiatry* **144**: 453–62

Whitton A, Appleby L, Warner R (1996) Maternal thinking and the treatment of postnatal depression. *Int Rev Psychiatry* **8**(1): 73–8

Yamashito H, Yoshidal K, Nakano H, Tashiro N (2000) Postnatal depression in Japanese women. Detecting the early onset of postnatal depression by closely monitoring the postpartum mood. *J Affect Disord* **58**(2): 145–54

10

Coping with loss and bereavement

Symbolically a baby represents the beginning of life and the ultimate in human creativity. A child symbolises innocence, vulnerability, pleasure and potential for growth. When any child dies, against the natural order of things, an important thread of continuity is broken.

(Hindmarch, 1994, p. 24)

In *Chapter 6,* we touched on the subject of loss, considering how women may respond to the changes that affect them at this stage of their life. When we considered loss in pregnancy we were focusing on changes that come about because of differences in lifestyle brought about by pregnancy. In this chapter the focus is on the experience of a much more concrete loss: the loss of a baby through miscarriage, stillbirth, termination or perinatal death.

We have probably all experienced loss in some way and at some time during our lives. Perhaps it is only a small personal item that suddenly cannot be found; a purse or an address book for example, or maybe some of us have experienced a more significant loss, such as the break up of a close relationship. Other people will have had to cope with a major loss because someone that they love has died. Whatever the loss, people seem to experience similar psychological states as they come to terms with what has happened to them. These stages are known as grieving, often described as the grieving process because people seem to go through a number of different stages before they are able to come to terms with what has happened to them.

The purpose of this chapter is twofold. Firstly, it helps the reader to understand the psychological mechanisms that come into play when parents cope with grieving for a lost baby. Whether this loss is caused through miscarriage, termination for fetal abnormality, stillbirth or neonatal loss, we consider some of the ways that parents may react following the death of their baby. As the quotation at the beginning of this chapter suggests, death of a baby runs counter to all our expectations of birth: we anticipate the entrance of a new life into the world with hope and pleasure; we look forward to seeing the baby grow and develop; we enjoy its youth. Death is the antithesis of this. In our minds we link death with the elderly, with infirmity and the conclusion of life, so it seems particularly sad and upsetting when a baby dies before it has even had a chance of life.

The second aim is to help you understand your own reactions to the death of a baby. Although as a midwife you are a professional who is 'trained' to deal with life and death situations, you will inevitably find it hard to handle the loss of a baby. After all, your job is about bringing life into the world, not losing it. If you have been present at the delivery or involved with the mother during the pregnancy you may wonder whether there was anything that you could have done to prevent the outcome. You may find it hard to know how to comfort the grieving parents as well as handling your own emotions. This chapter aims to give you suggestions on how you can deal with your own emotions and how to cope with the feelings of failure and sadness. The particular dilemma of the clash between the professional and personal will also be considered. The midwife may have experienced her own painful bereavements; whether through the death of an adult or baby and one's own emotions and memories can be triggered by the loss of another.

By the time you have finished reading this chapter you will have a better understanding of the process of grieving and be better able to assist parents who are dealing with loss. This might go some way to preventing the 'psychological morbidity' associated with the loss of a baby. However, this is not intended to be a crash course in counselling. It would not be possible to teach all the skills that you will need to use when you come into contact with bereaved families. It will try to give you some understanding of the psychological factors involved in grief and loss, so that you gain a deeper understanding of how families might react when their baby dies.

Types of loss

It is not my intention to discuss every possible kind of loss during pregnancy and the early postpartum, there are so many possibilities that it would not be possible to cover them all. Rather, I will talk about the concept of loss more generally and refer to specific kinds of loss that are most likely to affect midwifery practice. We will consider miscarriage, termination (for fetal abnormality), stillbirth, perinatal death. The support required for the parents of a baby requiring terminal care will not be discussed and neither will cot death. Although it is acknowledged that these are terrible losses, it is felt that these are more in the realms of neonatal/paediatric care, rather than midwifery care. We touch briefly on the ideas of loss of a 'perfect' baby, when we discuss how the midwife might help someone come to terms with the birth of a handicapped child.

What is loss?

As mentioned earlier, we have all experienced loss on many occasions, even if we have not experienced bereavement. Loss may be trivial, or it may be a life-changing experience. It may involve a physical object, such as a personal possession, or may involve a change in life, such as a change of job, of house or of school. Sometimes we are not always aware of losses because they are not acknowledged by society as being 'genuine losses'. In such cases we are often surprised when people become depressed and disorientated. *Chapter 9* discussed how some women may become depressed after giving birth because they are having to cope with a change in life and may be grieving for their past lifestyle. We have already discussed this concept in relation to pregnancy. Similarly, the adolescent starting a job or university may experience a sense of loss for the familiarity and relative security of school. In general, society sees these as positive changes in life and so often we do not understand our own feelings when coping with these situations.

Whatever the situation, reactions to loss will depend on the individual and on the importance of the object or event. To look at our previous examples, loss of a wallet that has almost nothing in it is likely to be less of a problem than a wallet containing valuable and sentimental items. Such an object cannot easily be replaced and its loss will cause quite a lot of trouble to the individual. In the same vein, loss of the security of school may be no problem to the young person who has always hated school, but require considerable readjustment for the adolescent who has enjoyed and valued their schooldays.

Despite these individual differences we can all empathise with feelings of loss. You may remember the panicky feelings when you thought you had lost an object of great sentimental value. You may also have experienced great anger if you have been burgled or have lost some prized possession. Although it is true that you cannot 'know' what a parent feels when they have lost a child, you should be able to recognise the emotions and understand them, albeit at a superficial level.

It is important to remember that loss is never an isolated event but brings in its wake many other losses. Consider the example of a man or woman losing their job; this in itself is hard to cope with, but it might also mean many other losses. If the job was important to the person's self-concept then there will be loss of identity. Loss of income will mean that valued activities might have to be given up. Loss of work companions will be another issue. In other words, losses lead to other losses and this is why the experience can be so devastating and require a long period of adjustment and recovery.

What is grief?

Grief is the psychological response to loss. It is, as Mander (1994) puts it, 'the other side of the coin' (p.16) of a loving relationship. It can also reflect a reaction to any other kind of loss. For example, it is possible to grieve for the loss of something other than a person. Niven (1992) points out that it is hard to be specific when talking about grief reactions. Every person is unique and will react in an individual way, but research into grief is necessarily limited. Research subjects are almost inevitably a self-selected sample as it would be ethically unacceptable to carry out research with unwilling subjects who were trying to cope with grief. The research sample cannot be described as typical of all people who have suffered loss or bereavement. Niven also reminds us that as people move on after bereavement to some sense of acceptance, they do not forget their loss. If a couple goes on to have another baby, or purchase some material object to love, such as a puppy, they do not forget the child they have lost.

How can we try and quantify a parent's love for their child? Similarly, how can we try and imagine the extent of their grief if that child dies? We cannot, of course, but we can and should attempt to understand some of the feelings associated with bereavement and understand our own complex reactions in order to provide the parents with constructive help.

Bereavement

Bereavement is a particular kind of loss that occurs when a close relative or friend dies. In this situation feelings of loss are intensified because the individual who has died can never be replaced. The loss is far more profound, deeper and more painful. It may raise anxieties about our own mortality and fear of death. Our sense of loss when we experience bereavement is hard to predict in terms of quantifiable measures, such as age or length of relationship (Stewart and Dent, 1994). Similarly in pregnancy, the sense of loss does not always equate with the gestation of the pregnancy. It is impossible to develop a 'hierarchy' of grief and loss, where a miscarriage at six weeks can be seen as 'less tragic' than a stillbirth at term; the depth and extent of the loss can only be defined by the individual. As one friend said to me when talking about her own miscarriage: she was mourning 'all those hopes and dreams'. On realising that she was pregnant she already felt a bond with her baby, thinking of it as a person with its whole life stretching ahead — to have that life taken away seemed cruelly unfair. Consider Bowlby's theorics of attachment and loss. The level of attachment may be equated with an equal feeling of loss if the baby dies. We cannot presume to know what a parent's attachment to the baby is, we also cannot presume to define or comprehend the extent of the loss.

What are the psychological responses to grief?

Research indicates that typical reactions to bereavement tend to be anger, restlessness and sadness (Niven, 1992). Niven suggests that it may be impossible for another individual to empathise with a parent's sense of loss unless they have had a similar experience. This is not to say that a midwife who has not experienced such a loss cannot offer constructive support — of course she can. It is important to recognise that some parents may only feel safe discussing the enormity of their loss with others who have had similar experiences. The loss of a child must cause tidal waves of emotion that, at times, seem very frightening. Parents may use all sorts of strategies to avoid these overpowering emotions. They may feel that they can discuss their feelings with other parents who have experienced the death of a child.

Kubler-Ross (1970) who carried out a lot of work with people who were terminally ill, suggested that there are five stages of grieving, namely: denial, anger, bargaining, depression and finally acceptance. A mother who has been told that her baby is stillborn may express denial and state that she can still feel it moving. Parents often experience denial when first told that their baby has died. One father writes:

> *I had no idea how to react. I felt so detached from the whole business. I gazed out of the window and cuddled Rosalind as she wept. It was almost that I was imagining the whole affair… As the end of the labour drew near, I nurtured a secret hope that they had all been wrong, that our baby would emerge alive and fighting for life.*

(Kohner and Henley, 1991 p. 31)

Denial: This seems to be a coping mechanism that we use unconsciously to protect us from the enormity of what has happened. We find it so difficult to understand the finality of death that it is impossible for us to react immediately. After hearing of a death people report a sense of numbness and unreality. A sense of 'this can't really be happening to me' and as the quotation above indicates, a hope that this is all some dreadful dream from which you will soon awaken to find everything as normal. People often go through their normal daily life, as if they were in a dream world. Suddenly normal, everyday things seem strange and unfamiliar when viewed in the context of the loss that someone has experienced.

Anger: This sometimes follows denial. People feel angry that the event has been allowed to happen. Sometimes they feel angry with the person who has died, sometimes they feel angry with themselves, sometimes they feel anger towards the people who have been caring for their loved-one in the time leading up to the death. Commonly, parents describe this anger as being almost violent in nature — some parents express a wish to be able to physically lash out, or to hit something. Borg and Lasker (1982) suggest that women may find it harder than men to express their anger and may suffer deeper depression as a result. While anger can be a healthy emotion it can be very damaging if the couple then direct their anger at each other.

Mander (1994) noted the problems that can arise when the anger is directed at health professionals. As part of her research she asked midwives how they felt when faced with a grieving parent's anger. The midwives all acknowledged that anger was a part of the grieving process and coped by reminding themselves that the anger was not directed at them in person. As Mander comments, this is another emotional demand placed on the midwife: that of coping with another's anger without responding to that anger in any way.

Bargaining: This is most likely to happen in situations before a death has occurred, when people feel that they may be able to avert the inevitable crisis. It takes the form of: 'If only you will let X live, then I will...'. Very often people turn to God or some higher-being for this bargaining. This stage of the grieving process may occur when parents are told that the child they are expecting has some kind of abnormality, or might also occur when miscarriage or stillbirth is threatened. In short, it may happen in any situation where there is still some hope of life and/or normality. It is almost as if people are trying to bring the situation back under their own control. By offering to do something, or change some aspect of their personality, they hope to change the course of history and avert the horrors of the loss.

Depression: This stage usually follows the stages of denial and bargaining as people slowly come to terms with what has happened to them. Gradually, the reality of the situation sinks in with the realisation that events cannot be changed. The baby is dead: the miscarriage has happened; the perfect child that was hoped for is damaged. In this stage, parents may feel an overwhelming sense of sadness and hopelessness. Life might appear entirely black with no rays of sunshine on the horizon. People might experience uncontrollable periods of weeping, or even anger. There is often a sense of, 'Why me/us? What did we do to deserve this? Why have other people been able to produce normal and healthy babies?' Sometimes parents will feel that they are being punished for something that they have done wrong in the past. This is a very bleak time for people.

It is almost impossible to say how long this part of the grieving process will last, or with what intensity. There is no easy way of predicting. For example, it might be argued that a woman who has had a miscarriage at six weeks' gestation should grieve less than a woman who has carried a baby to term and has had a stillbirth. However, much will depend on several other factors. While it may be true that the woman who did not intend to get pregnant, might be relieved at having a miscarriage, for the woman who has been trying to conceive for years, the experience could be devastating.

Acceptance: The final stage of the grieving process according to Kubler-Ross is acceptance. Acceptance is seen as a sense of resignation to what has happened. It is not necessarily a 'happy outcome' or 'coming to terms', although it could be both of these things. Perhaps it would be true to say that people are more likely to overcome and come to terms with a miscarriage, than the loss of a baby at term. But even as I write this, I am aware of two friends, one of whom experienced a miscarriage and the other whose baby died shortly after birth. I know that both of these women think about the child they lost and keep a mental record of the age that the child would have been if they had lived. Indeed, my own mother had an ectopic pregnancy when I was eight years old, and I have often wondered how different my life would have been had I had a younger brother or sister. Acceptance is simply the stage at which you start getting on with life again.

The stages of grief as they have been described above are a useful way of understanding what might be happening to someone after they have experienced a major loss. It is important not to be too prescriptive about these and it would be entirely wrong to assume that everyone goes through all the stages in the same order. There may be some who do not feel angry or feel the need to bargain. People may miss out some stages, or go back to previous stages. They may go through some stages very quickly, and get stuck in others. As Mander (1994) points out, professionals need to be wary of 'expecting' the process of grief to follow a pattern. The concept of stages of grief is useful in emphasising the dynamic and changing nature of grieving, but should not be used by the midwife to try and 'second-guess' what the parents will experience next. The fact that they are apparently denying the death of their baby now, does not mean that they will automatically start to feel angry next.

Hindmarch (1994) also points out that describing grief as a process with different stages can be fraught with difficulty. No two people will react in the same way to the same loss: just as each baby's birth is unique, so each parent's response to the death of a baby will be particular to them. One mother is quoted as saying:

> *Don't talk to me about the grieving process... What a ludicrously inappropriate phrase to define the mental, physical and emotional turmoil you are left to sort out after your child has died.*

(Hindmarch, 1994, p. 23)

Cognitive processes in psychological adaptation to loss

The stages of grief that have been described above seem to be very much linked with emotional reactions to the experience. Some authors have concentrated more on the rational, thinking processes that have to change if parents are going to be able to cope with their loss. The cognitive processes in psychological adaptation refer to the processes by which parents come to 'know' or understand the extent of their loss, in other words, how parents adjust to their bereavement. Taylor (1983) describes three steps in this process of adaptation, namely:

❖ A search for meaning (an understanding of the event).

❖ A search for mastery (development of control over the event or its recurrence).

❖ A search for self-enhancement (an attempt to counteract the fall in self-esteem consequent upon a negative event) (quoted in Tunaley *et al*, 1993, p. 370.).

Grief can be described as the reaction to a bereavement, while mourning is what one does to express grief (Hindmarch, 1994). Rajan and Oakley (1993) comment on the 'vital process' (p. 75) of mourning but note that in Western society the loss of a baby may not be given the level of social significance that legitimates mourning. As a result parents may try to hide their feelings, or may think that they are being 'silly' and 'self-indulgent'. They may begin to wonder whether they have a problem, or even whether they are going mad. They may, however, be afraid to discuss these concerns with anyone for they may feel that no one will understand. Rajan and Oakley (1993) extrapolated information from their study on social support in pregnancy to ascertain the importance of social support for women who had suffered pregnancy loss. One of the most staggering findings of this study is only mentioned in passing. Forty-three per cent of the 509 women enrolled in the study had previously had one or more pregnancy losses. It is true that women who enrolled in the study had to have a history of at least one low birth weight baby so they were not a 'typical' group of pregnant women. Nonetheless, this underlines the frequency with which pregnancy loss occurs. It is not a 'rare event' that warrants little attention. Many women are affected and their experience of loss will inevitably influence their feelings about future pregnancies. Rajan and Oakley stress that it is necessary to allow women to decide what form social support should take, responding to her individual needs and not attempting to be directive in any way.

Grief and the midwife

How can the midwife offer help and yet protect her own needs? Healthcare professionals used to be admonished for becoming too involved with clients and their families. However, now things are a little different. Stewart and Dent (1994) point out that while it is acceptable to cry with a client 'the tears should be for their pain and suffering and not ours' (p. 5). This is all very well, but how can you become involved in a positive fashion while protecting yourself from pain? Larson (1993) uses the metaphor of the helper's pit to describe the difference between constructive and unconstructive help. Imagine that the person you wish to help is stuck at the bottom of a pit while you are at the edge of the pit. If you identify too closely with that person's problems you will fall into the pit with them. To help that person in a more constructive way, you need to be able to offer more positive help. To use another analogy, the helper can show empathy and understanding by throwing a rope ladder down into the pit and helping the person to climb out.

The midwife may indeed feel grief and it is not wrong to weep over the death of a baby. However, her grief is hers, and cannot be compared to the grief felt by the woman and her family. Similarly, it is not wrong if the midwife does not show any overt grief— this does not infer that she is any better or worse than the midwife who weeps. Research by Moulder (1998) indicates that not all women want to be faced with the midwife's own emotions. Spall and Callis (1997) point out that the guiding principle should be that the professional, in this case the midwife, is there for the woman and her family and not vice versa. The midwife's own need for sympathy and support might be very acute, but her colleagues, family and friends should meet these needs. It is vital that midwives have their own support network so that they can care for their own well being.

Attachment to the fetus

It is important at this point to say something about attachment to the fetus because this does have some bearing on how women respond to perinatal loss. It has been noted that there is quite considerable variation in when women report that they begin to feel an attachment to their unborn child. For some, it seems to happen right from the beginning. Almost as soon as a woman knows that she is pregnant she feels a bond with her baby to be. For other women a sense of attachment does not occur until quickening or when they see the first scan. It is only then that the fetus becomes a 'real person' to them. There are other women who do not feel a bond with their baby until after the birth, when the baby has become a reality. It seems that all these ways of responding are normal, and they are not related to the relationship that a mother will ultimately develop with her baby once he or she is born. The time of attachment does have a bearing on how a woman responds to loss of pregnancy. A miscarriage at twelve weeks may not be that distressing to the woman who has no sense of her babies' presence and feels no attachment, whereas it will inevitably be a more distressing experience for the woman who has felt attached to her baby from the moment of discovering her pregnancy.

Linked with attachment to the fetus is the concept of the fantasy baby. Probably most parents have a concept of what the baby will be like when he or she is eventually born. This concept is the 'fantasy baby' because it is only a projection of the physical and psychological characteristics of the child-to-be. As yet, there is no reality against which to test it. Again, individuals vary in how much they invest in the fantasy baby, with some people having much clearer and firmer ideas of what the baby will be like than others. At birth, almost all parents will have to give up their concept of the fantasy baby and come to know the real baby. This may be particularly difficult for parents whose child is not perfect at birth, who has, for example, to go into the special care baby unit, or who is born with some defect. For the child who is stillborn or who dies in the first few days after birth, they may remain as the fantasy baby and always be idealised as having been perfect. This may have consequences for subsequent children born to the parents who can never match up to the perfect baby image that the parents have projected on to the lost child (see *pp. 250–251*).

Different kinds of loss in pregnancy and the postpartum

Having looked more generally at the grief process, we will now concentrate on the specific kinds of loss that a person could encounter during pregnancy and the early postpartum. We begin with miscarriage, because that seems the logical place to begin, and then go on to discuss abortion for fetal abnormality, stillbirth and neonatal death.

Miscarriage

This may occur at a time when few people may know that the woman is pregnant. She will have received none of the public admiration that she may have gained had her 'bump' started to grow and become noticeable. She may feel cheated of this recognition of her pregnancy. She may also receive little sympathy for the miscarriage and be expected to get over it quickly and get back to work. She may be told that it is 'nature's way', implying that she has created an abnormal and imperfect child (Stewart and Dent, 1994, p.16).

Miscarriage is also unusual because in many ways it could be argued that women are grieving for a 'potential child' rather than a real child. This may have the effect of making grieving more complicated and less easy to overcome. With miscarriage there is no body to mourn, no concrete proof that the life was ever real and genuine. For many women this will make the loss more difficult to manage, particularly when society at large does not acknowledge the full extent of her grief. It has been suggested that women who have a miscarriage are less likely to receive appropriate attention and support than women who have a stillbirth or neonatal death (Friedman and Cohen, 1982). I suspect that this is because it is not generally accepted that miscarriage constitutes a real loss.

Tunaley *et al* (1993) suggest that, 'the cognitions surrounding miscarriage are certainly poorly documented' (p. 370). In an attempt to overcome this lack of knowledge the authors interviewed twenty-two women some months after their first miscarriage. Although this is a small and self-selected sample, the results are thought-provoking. Nineteen of the women (86%) had arrived at one or more explanations for their miscarriage: these included a belief that a medical problem was the cause, stress, self-miscarriage or God's punishment.

These feelings of guilt and self-blame are interesting: why do women blame themselves? Is this something to do with societal pressures that infer that all the problems of the child are the mother's fault? Or is it simply that women find it easier to blame themselves rather than some anonymous outside party. Although most of the women (81%) stated that they would make changes to their lifestyle in future pregnancies, few thought that this would actually achieve anything — that is, women felt that they had little mastery over events. Half of the women appeared to use self-enhancement as a coping strategy. They saw themselves as 'better off' than others in a similar situation. Some saw themselves as lucky that the miscarriage had not occurred later in pregnancy, whereas others considered themselves fortunate that they already had children. These downward comparisons did not make any significant difference in helping women to adjust to their loss.

In another study, Cecil (1994) looked at women's views of care following miscarriage. Fifty women in Northern Ireland who had had no more than two miscarriages were interviewed first in hospital following the miscarriage; then two to three weeks later; then approximately three months after the first contact with a final interview six months after the miscarriage. While I acknowledge that midwives rarely have contact with women in hospital immediately following miscarriage, the results are nonetheless important for midwifery practice. These suggested that most of the women in the sample did not feel that they had received an adequate service. They felt that information and explanation was lacking, as were some aspects of hospital care and aftercare. They also felt that the health professionals with whom they came into contact did not fully understand or acknowledge the full extent of their loss. A finding echoed in a study carried out in England by Prettyman and Cordle (1992) and in a number of more recent studies discussed below.

Similar to the study referred to earlier by Tunaley *et al*, women in Cecil's sample tried to put the miscarriage into some sort of context and make sense of it. Although Cecil does not explore this theme in any great detail, it is apparent that some women in her study felt a sort of fatalism — that the 'control' of the miscarriage was out of their hands. As Cecil points out, miscarriage may be a woman's first experience of bereavement. As was discussed in the chapter on birth, women now have fewer children and, with social and demographic changes, may have little experience of birth until they experience it for themselves. Similarly, improvements in health ensure that most people now reach adulthood with little or no experience of bereavement. How do they cope when they have had so little preparation and when death remains a taboo subject? And, particularly when the loss is of a baby — a death that confounds all our beliefs in the normal passage of life? Cecil suggests that women who have a miscarriage do not expect hospital staff to share their grief but do expect to be treated with care and sympathy. I think that this is an important point. Women expressed a need for explanation and discussion; such discussion seems to help prevent feelings of guilt.

In her study, Cecil found that most women had little or no contact with health professionals following discharge from hospital, and for many women this was a source of dissatisfaction. Women who contacted their GP were sometimes disappointed with their response, eg. one woman was simply offered antidepressants. Many women who have a first trimester miscarriage may not even have had their booking appointment with the midwife but perhaps there is a place for the midwife to contact all women who have had a miscarriage, whether or not they have met previously to provide a 'listening service'. This may seem an unrealistic suggestion given the heavy workload of most midwives — but, if this is a service that has the potential to prevent psychological morbidity then it might be worth considering. Such a service would at least provide tangible acknowledgment to the woman that she has lost a baby — a real person with whom she has had a unique attachment. Cecil claims that although health professionals may be very concerned about the care of women who have miscarried, this concern is often not apparent to the woman herself. She suggests that the workload needs to be organised to enable health professionals to make more time available to women who have had a miscarriage.

Studies carried out in North America by Brier (1999) and in France by Garel *et al* (1994) highlight the importance of patient debriefing following miscarriage. Both studies surveyed patient satisfaction following a miscarriage and found that there was a lot of anger and dissatisfaction with the medical care received. Brier's sample reported that physician's tended to be generally insensitive to the loss the woman had experienced. Satisfaction was greatest when there was a follow-up appointment shortly after the loss where the woman could discuss issues about why the miscarriage had happened and whether it was likely to occur again. Brier also found that in the majority of women feelings of loss characterised by grief, dysphoria and anxiety were short-lived. Women tended to feel more distress if:

- it was a strongly desired pregnancy
- it had taken a long time to conceive
- there were no other living children
- they had had elective abortions in the past
- there had been no warning signs that the miscarriage was likely to occur
- the loss was relatively late in the pregnancy
- they had little social support and a past history of coping badly with difficult situations.

In these cases depressive and anxiety disorders tended to continue accompanied by worries about future reproductive competence.

A study by Robinson *et al* (1994) also highlights those women who are likely to take longer to recover from a miscarriage. This team undertook a longitudinal study of seventy Canadian women who had experienced a miscarriage. Women who participated were asked to complete questionnaires at three months, six months and one year after their loss. Fourteen women (41.2%) felt that the miscarriage was partly their fault. These women were significantly more likely to show higher depression scores one year after the event. The research also showed that young women and those who already had children were no less likely to be depressed following miscarriage than older nulliparous women. It is wrong to assume that simply because a woman appears to have ample opportunity to become pregnant again, that she will get over the miscarriage any faster than another woman. As Robinson *et al* point out, health workers need to be wary of making any assumptions about how a woman may react to miscarriage. While the term 'precious pregnancy' is often given to women who are pregnant following fertility treatment or following previous pregnancy loss, it cannot be assumed that a woman pregnant for the eighth time, with seven healthy children does not feel her pregnancy to be equally precious. It is arguable that input from the midwife or another professional following the miscarriage might prevent these feelings of loss and subsequent depression.

Termination for fetal abnormality

As the law stands in Britain at the moment, elective terminations of pregnancy can be carried out legally if two or more medical practitioners agree that:

❖ The pregnancy has not continued for longer than twenty-four weeks, and continuation of it would cause risk of injury to the physical or mental health of the mother or other children in the family.

❖ Termination has to take place in order to prevent permanent damage to the physical or mental health of the mother.

❖ The woman's life would be at risk if the pregnancy continues.

❖ There is a substantial risk that if the child is born it will be seriously disabled.

There are obviously enormous ethical issues that surround the debate on abortion. Legal arguments quickly become confused and tied up in moral and religious debates about the sanctity of life, and the complexity of these arguments often make it difficult to think clearly about the issue of termination of pregnancy. For this reason, this chapter discusses only those abortions that take place because of the woman's life being at risk and risk of severe fetal abnormality. While I appreciate that even these situations are not free of arguments of a moral nature, I feel that the situation in these conditions is more clear-cut and therefore more justifiable. Even if you object to abortion on religious or ethical grounds, most reasonable people can see that there is an argument for not allowing a woman to die during birth and for limiting the suffering that a handicapped child might experience if they are born. It is also easier to look at loss in this context too. There is evidence to suggest that women who have a termination of pregnancy for what might be described as more 'social' reasons appear to recover well from the experience (Clare and Tyrell, 1994). This is not to suggest that these women will not subsequently have problems, but at least in the short term, they manage to make a reasonably clear-cut decision about their future. The situation is qualitatively different for those parents who have to make an agonising decision to terminate a pregnancy because the baby is abnormal or the mother's life is at risk

According to Mander (1994) the rate of termination for fetal abnormality is fairly constant: about 1–2% are undertaken before the pregnancy has reached twenty weeks; around 17% are carried out after this time. A woman's decision to have a termination if a baby she is carrying is found to have abnormalities probably begins to form even before she decides to become pregnant.

Moulder (1998) found that in her study of women's experiences of termination, there were clear phases in the decision-making process. Firstly, there was the realisation of the pregnancy; this was closely followed by the decision to go ahead with the termination. This decision was in some cases made alone, in others with the help of a partner, friend or professional. Other stages involved the arrangement of the termination, the termination itself and finally, the period of reflection following the termination. The women who took part in the study felt that they had to jump through a number of hurdles to arrange the termination. It was a difficult decision to make and they were anxious because they thought that others might judge them unfavourably. Several women felt that they had made a decision without having spoken of it properly to anyone. Having said this, there were differences in the way that the women in the study reacted, some making the decision far more easily than others. This finding highlights the importance of recognising that it is not possible to make generalised statements about women's reactions to a termination. For some it will be a relief, for others an agonising decision.

There are similarities between miscarriage and stillbirth because parents have to come to terms with the loss of a child. However, unlike miscarriage or stillbirth, in a termination the parents have to cope with the added stress of having to decide actively to end their baby's life. Even though this decision might well be made with the best interests of the baby at heart and in some cases will be clearer than others, it is nevertheless a decision that takes a great deal of courage and one that needs to be treated sympathetically by others. As one midwife in Moulder's study commented:

> *Usually it is a wanted baby and it's a baby that is alive and well, albeit with some abnormality and the parents are having to make the decision to actively end the pregnancy. So basically they are terminating the baby's life as it were... with a stillbirth, yes it is a wanted baby and its died but it's beyond your control.*

(Moulder, 1998, p. 103)

The difficulty in making such a life-changing decision is highlighted in a small-scale qualitative study by Bryar (1997). Women in this study made the point that the decision was the hardest thing they ever did leading the researcher to conclude that, 'the decision to interrupt a pregnancy is a profound experience that permeates all areas of a woman's life' (p. 559).

Although there has been no systematic research on the topic, I suspect that the later in pregnancy a termination is carried out the more difficult is the decision and the greater the distress felt by those making the decision. This is certainly a perception shared by a number of health professionals. Some of these also commented that it was difficult to know how to approach women who had had a termination late in pregnancy (Moulder, 1998).

Stillbirth

Broadly speaking, we can talk of two kinds of stillbirth: those that are 'known' because the mother has become aware that the baby she is carrying has died and those that are unexpected because an otherwise healthy child dies during birth (Mander, 1994). It is perhaps tempting to think that an 'expected' stillbirth is somehow less traumatic than one that is unexpected, because the parents can at least begin the process of grieving, but in reality this is probably not the case. Both are equally shocking and distressing because most couples anticipate the birth of a healthy baby. To find that this is not the case inevitably requires major psychological readjustment.

Mander (1994) points out the devastating nature of the distress a woman may feel to learn that the baby she is carrying is dead. Some women are appalled at the thought and see themselves as a sort of 'living coffin' (Raphael-Leff, 1991), others may feel that their own body has somehow 'let the baby down'. Once it is known that a stillbirth is inevitable a decision has to be made about when to induce birth. The key here probably lies in listening to the woman herself. Some will want to get the birth over and done with as quickly as possible, whereas others may wish to wait for a day or so (always assuming that this is medically possible). Women must be helped to understand the changes that are likely to take place in the fetus, the longer they wait to give birth. They may also have to cope with a long and painful labour, that produces nothing but a dead child. All of this is extremely difficult for people to cope with, professionals as well as parents. Moulder (1998) found in her study that professionals often had not had many experiences of coping with a stillbirth. Many had had numerous dealings with miscarriage in the early stages of pregnancy, but had not experienced late termination of pregnancy or stillbirth, therefore for them it was a relatively rare event and they did not necessarily feel that they had the skills to deal with the parents.

Perinatal death

In many ways this seems the worst kind of perinatal loss that parents might have to endure. To have gone through a pregnancy, given birth to a live baby and then have to cope with its death shortly afterwards must be agonising for parents. I am sure that some people who have had this experience never fully recover from the memory. The way a perinatal death is handled by the midwife and other professionals can ease the pain for the parents to a certain extent. This is discussed more fully in the next section.

The consequences of perinatal loss

There is an accumulating body of evidence that perinatal loss leads to enhanced anxiety about subsequent pregnancies. Depression is also a common consequence. Nearly all studies report similar findings, although level of anxiety experienced and recovery from grief seems to vary according to a number of different factors, like the number of losses experienced and the time that has elapsed since the loss. Inevitably, a pregnancy that follows perinatal loss will be accompanied by more negative emotions than a pregnancy uncomplicated by such experiences. Franche and Mikail (1999) carried out a study in which the emotional adjustment of pregnant couples with and without a history of perinatal loss were compared. The group included thirty-one pregnant women who had experienced perinatal loss (PL) and thirty-one women who had a normal pregnancy history. Twenty-eight men in the PL group and twenty-three in the control group were also included. Unsurprisingly, couples in the PL group reported more symptoms that were related to depression and anxiety.

Cote-Arsenault and Marshall (2000) found that pregnancy following a pregnancy loss was laden with anxiety and lacking in joy. These authors carried out a qualitative study of thirteen women who were aged from twenty-four to forty-two years. The women reported that in a subsequent pregnancy there was a tendency to relive the past. They also found it difficult to live with wavering expectations of the new pregnancy. Although these women tried to stay balanced and accept this as a different pregnancy, they reported that the pregnancy felt like 'weathering the storm' and expecting the worst.

It can be seen from the studies reported so far that recent research has looked at reactions of both mothers and fathers to pregnancy loss. While both partners experience feelings of sadness, most studies report gender differences in what helps to alleviate the feelings of grief and anxiety (Ride, 1998). Several studies have now focused on fathers' reactions to perinatal loss (Wagner *et al*, 1997). A study carried out in Australia by Conway and Russell (2000) found that following a miscarriage, male partners experienced more feelings of sadness than their partners. Unlike their female partners, these men did not find social support particularly helpful in enabling them to come to terms with their loss. Murray *et al* (2000) found that higher levels of education were linked with lower levels of parental distress. They also found that the mothers in their sample recovered better if they felt that they had many friends in whom they could confide. Rich (2000) studied a sample of 249 bereaved mothers and 114 of their partners. The participants had experienced from one to twelve pregnancy losses at a gestational age of between two and forty-two weeks. In this study the significant predictors of grief outcome among the mothers were months since the loss, whether the individuals had attended counselling and attendance at support groups. For the fathers significant factors were the length of the pregnancy, talking with friends and talking with the family.

In general, women seem to find the social support of friends particularly helpful in coming to terms with pregnancy loss. This seems to be true for losses that occur at any time either during pregnancy or after the birth of the child. Engler and Lasker (2000) looked at a sample of mothers who had experienced a newborn death. In the year following the bereavement seventy-five mothers were interviewed. The results indicated that perceived support and emotion-focused coping were the factors that accounted for 43% of the variance in the grief experienced. In other words, women who felt that they had enough support and who focused on their feelings about the bereavement seemed to cope better than other women. The authors of this study concluded that programmes to help bereaved mothers to find support and explore different ways of coping would be beneficial in helping them to cope successfully with their loss.

Pregnancy loss can also have consequences for subsequent children born to couples, although findings are not always consistent and caution should be used when interpreting the results. Generally speaking, it seems as if some parents have difficulty in adapting to the 'replacement child', especially if the new baby arrives before the parents have properly grieved for their loss. Explanations for this finding suggest that the child that was lost remains a perfect fantasy and no real-child can ever live up to this ideal which has an impact on the mother-infant and father-infant relationship. Heller and Zeanah (1999) studied a group of mothers who had had another child within nineteen months of losing a baby. They assessed mother-infant attachment when the babies were twelve months old and found that 45% of the sample demonstrated disorganised attachment to their mothers. This result was significantly higher than the expected rate of 15% found in other middle-class samples. There is some evidence to suggest that difficulties with attachment could begin in the ante-natal period. Armstrong and Hutti (1998) looked at a group of thirty-one women. Fifteen were in their first pregnancy. The remaining sixteen had all experienced a late miscarriage, stillbirth or neonatal death. Armstrong looked at both anxiety and prenatal attachment and found that women who had experienced a perinatal loss were not only more anxious but also less attached to the baby they were now carrying. Such unwillingness to become attached to the new baby is understandable, as parents are undoubtedly shielding themselves from the pain of another potential loss. Unfortunately, this protective mechanism might have a negative impact on the mother's relationship with her new baby.

Not all studies report such negative findings. Gout and Romanoff (2000) found that parents adapted to their losses in different ways, many of which were very positive. They often emphasised the importance of parenting subsequent children, but maintained the connection to the dead child through storytelling. Parents also tended to preserve a space in the family that the dead child would have inhabited. The families in this study seemed to make a better adjustment to their loss and subsequent children were not reported as suffering.

Implications for practice

Over a period of twenty years or so there have been enormous changes in the way professionals handle miscarriage, stillbirth and neonatal death. In the main these changes are in a positive direction, and there is a growing recognition that parents needs must be taken into account. Whereas at one time, little attention was paid to the psychological effects of early miscarriage, there is now an understanding that this might represent a very significant life event for some couples. It was once common practice to remove a stillborn baby and dispose of it, so that the mother would not be upset at the appearance of the dead baby, but now parents are encouraged to see the baby and perhaps take photographs as a memento. The infant is given a proper funeral, so that parents can say farewell and acknowledge their loss. These changes to practice have taken place partly because of the views expressed by parents themselves and partly because of a better understanding of the psychological processes that take place during grieving. It is well recognised that grief is less likely to become complicated if an individual has a concrete entity to grieve for. It is easier for parents to mourn their dead child if they know what it looks like than for something that they have never seen. Even if the baby is deformed it is probably better for the parents to confront this, rather than imagining something worse.

Having said all of this, I sometimes feel concerned that there is a prevailing attitude that to cuddle and photograph your dead baby is seen as 'good' whereas not wanting to do this is seen as 'bad'. In reality there will inevitably be wide individual differences in what people find helpful. Some parents will want to spend long hours with their dead baby, others may not find this helpful at all and should not be put under pressure to do things because that is the present 'trend'. There may be some who will not want to see the baby at first, and it may take several days before they can bring themselves to confront their loss. Health professionals should try not to be prescriptive about what is 'best' for people, instead they need to listen to parents and help them grieve for their loss in whatever way is best for them, accepting that all of us are individuals. There is not a right and wrong way to grieve. Many people will need to cry and may find an outward expression of emotion helpful; others may find such a loss of control makes them feel even worse. Stereotyping is not helpful; people have their own coping strategies that need to be considered and should be allowed to grieve in whatever way is best for them.

Death is never easy to cope with, particularly in modern society where we do not often come face-to-face with it. It is particularly difficult to help grieving parents because it is hard to know what will help them most. Some writers have suggested that it is acceptable for professionals to express their own emotions when dealing with difficult situations but I am not 100% convinced that this is appropriate in every case. The main role for the professional is to support the grieving parents; you certainly do not want to break down so that parents feel that they have to support you. Somehow you have to put your own needs into the background, you may well feel like breaking down and weeping, but you have to ask yourself whether this show of emotion will simply distress the parents even more. There are no hard and fast rules. Some parents might well find it helpful to see a midwife crying, it might make it easier for them to express their own grief and it may make them feel that the midwife truly empathises with their feelings. Others might feel angry; after all, it is not you who has just lost a child. A lot will depend on the relationship that you have with the parents, and the kind of person that you are as well as the circumstances surrounding the loss.

Perhaps the only way of dealing with the delicacy of the situation is to be as genuine as possible and for the midwife to try to be responsive to the situation. Listen to what the people you are dealing with are saying; give them time to express their needs. Do not make assumptions about what you think would be good for them. This means that you will have to be flexible and respond in different ways to different people. You also need to be reflective in your practice, constantly modifying your behaviour to respond to the needs of others. Of course, this is easier said than done, especially when you also have to cope with your own distress.

Another aspect of bereavement that the midwife has to be sensitively aware of is cultural differences. It is not within the scope of this book to deal with these cultural differences in detail.

However, it is obvious that it is crucially important to be sensitive to the needs of those from other cultures and to try to be aware of different practices that may seem odd or alien to you. Herbert (1998) points out that over the past twenty years practices for dealing with perinatal loss have changed dramatically. These practices are based on Euro-American theories of grief and loss that may not be appropriate for those from ethnic minority groups.

To some extent your knowledge of cultural differences in responding to grief and loss will depend upon the geographical area where you practice. Some midwives will not come into contact with women from ethnic minority groups while others will have many dealings with women from other cultures. If this is the case, then I feel that it is the midwife's responsibility to find out as much as possible about the way in which these cultures cope with death and dying so that she can respond appropriately if and when the need arises.

References

Armstrong D, Hutti M (1998) Pregnancy after perinatal loss: the relationship between anxiety and prenatal attachment. *J Obstet Gynecol Neonatal Nurs* 27(2): 183–9

Borg S, Lasker J (1982) *When Pregnancy Fails*. Routledge, London

Brier N (1999) Understanding and managing the emotional reactions to miscarriage. *Obstet Gynecol* 93(1): 151–5

Bryar SH (1997) One day you're pregnant and one day you're not: pregnancy interruption for fetal anomalies. *J Obstet Gynecol Neonatal Nurs* 26(5): 559–66

Cecil R (1994) Miscarriage: women's views of care. *J Reprod Infant Psychol* 12: 21–9

Clare AN, Tyrrell J (1994) Psychiatric aspects of abortion. *Irish J Psychological Med* 11: 92–8

Conway K, Russell G (2000) Couples' grief and experience of support in the aftermath of miscarriage. *Br J Med Psychol* 73(4): 531–45

Cote-Arsenault D, Marshall R (2000) One foot in — one foot out: weathering the storm of pregnancy after perinatal loss. *Res Nurs Health* 23(6): 473–85

Engler AJ, Lasker JN (2000) Predictors of maternal grief in the year after a newborn death. *Illness, Crisis and Loss* 8(3): 227–43

Franche RL, Mikail SF (1999) The impact of perinatal loss on adjustment to subsequent pregnancy. *Soc Sci Med* 48(11): 1613–23

Friedman R, Cohen KA (1982) Emotional reactions to the miscarriage of a consciously desired pregnancy. In: Notman MT, Nadelson C, eds. *The Woman Patient: Aggression, Adaptation and Psychotherapy*. Vol 3. Plenum Press, New York

Garel M, Blondel B, Lelong N, Bonenfant S, Kaminski M (1994) Long-term consequences of miscarriage: the depressive disorders and the following pregnancy. *J Reprod Infant Psychol* **12**: 233–40

Gout LA, Romanoff BD (2000) The myth of the replacement child: Parent's stories and practices after perinatal death. *Death Stud* **24**(2): 93–113

Herbert MP (1998) Perinatal bereavement in its cultural context. *Death Stud* **22**(1): 61–78

Hindmarch C (1994) *On the Death of a Child*. Radcliffe Medical Press, Oxford

Kohner M, Henley A (1992) *When a Baby Dies: The experience of late miscarriage, stillbirth and neonatal death*. Pandora Press, London

Kubler-Ross E (1970) *On Death and Dying*. Tavistock, London

Larson DG (1993) *The Helper's Journey: Working with people facing grief, loss and life threatening illness*. Research Press, Illinois

Maunder R (1994) *Loss and Bereavement in Childbearing*. Blackwell Scientific, Oxford

Moulder C (1998) *Understanding Pregnancy Loss: Perspectives and issues in care*. Macmillan, London

Murray JA, Terry DJ, Vance JC, Battistutta D, Connolly Y (2000) Effects of a program of intervention on parental distress following infant death. *Death Stud* **24**(4): 275–305

Niven CA (1992) *Physiological Care for Families before, during and after Birth*. Butterworth-Heinemann, Oxford

Prettyman RJ, Cordle CJ (1992) Psychological aspects of miscarriage: attitudes of the primary health care team. *Br J Gen Pract* **42**: 97–9

Rajan L, Oakley A (1993) No pills for the heartache: the importance of social support for women who suffer pregnancy loss. *J Reprod Infant Psychol* **11**: 25–87

Raphael-Leff J (1991) *Psychological Processes of Childbearing*. Chapman and Hall, London

Ride H (1998) Perinatal death: how fathers grieve. *MIDIRS Midwifery Digest* **8**(2): 242

Rich DE (2000) The impact of pregnancy loss services on grief outcome. Integrating research and practice in the design of perinatal bereavement programmes. *Illness, Crisis and Loss* **8**(3): 244–64

Robinson GE, Stirtzinger, R, Stewart DE, Ralecski M (1994) Psychological reactions in women followed for one year after miscarriage. *J Reprod Infant Psychol* **12**(1): 31–6

Spall B, Callis S (1997) *Loss, Bereavement and Grief: A guide to effective caring*. Stanley Thornes, Cheltenham

Stewart A, Dent A (1994) *At a Loss: Bereavement care when a baby dies*. Baillière Tindall, London

Taylor SE (1983) Adjustment to threatening events: a theory of cognitive adaptation. *Am Psychologist* **38**: 1161–73

Tunaley JR, Slade P, Duncan SB (1993) Cognitive processes in psychological adaptation to miscarriage: a preliminary report. *Psychol Health* **8**(3): 369–81

Wagner T, Higgins PG, Wallerstedt C (1997) Perinatal death: how fathers grieve. *J Perinat Educ* **6**(4): 9–16

Final word

This book came into existence for two reasons. There was not a text book on the market that brought together in one volume areas of psychology that seemed to me to be particularly relevant to midwifery practice and because of the midwifery students I taught. Over many years these women (and one or two men) inspired me by responding positively to the subject and helping me to see ways of making psychology applicable to midwifery settings. I felt that my teaching was very much a two-way process. I shared my knowledge of psychology and the midwives shared their understanding of the challenges they faced in their day-to-day interactions with others. The result was that we all learned together.

I hope that you have enjoyed reading the book and have found the contents accessible, challenging and relevant to your work as a midwife. I am aware that it has not been possible to cover all areas of psychology that would be of interest to midwives. I trust that I have covered enough topics to give the reader a broad understanding of relevant aspects of the subject and perhaps an interest to find out more.

The book will have served its purpose if you can see the relevance of psychology to your professional practice and use some of the theories in your day-to-day interactions with mothers and other professionals. I know that there are no easy answers contained in its pages but I hope that it will have helped you to become more aware of the complexity of social situations and of how your role can be influential. I hope that it will help you to recognise that people need to be seen as individuals and treated as such. In raising awareness of this perhaps you will be empowered to become more reflective in your practice and more aware of how you can influence situations so that over a period your professional skills are enhanced.

These comments about enhancing professional practice are not intended to be critical of midwives. In all my dealings with them both as a teacher of psychology and as a mother when I had my own children, I have found them to be sensitive and caring and supremely professional. I also know that midwives are passionate about their own continuing professional development. The contents of the book are offered to students of midwifery and practising midwives as an aid to help you to see your way through social complexity and to inform your practice. I hope that you will accept the contents in this light.

Ruth Paradice
March, 2002

Index